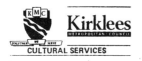

Kirklees
METROPOLITAN COUNCIL

CULTURAL SERVICES

Cultural Services Headquarter
Red Doles Lane,
Huddersfield. West Yorks. HI

writer. He is the author of eighteen popular medical and
science books and has also written extensively on medical
topics for *Reader's Digest* and *Good Housekeeping* books.
He has made many radio broadcasts and has appeared on
television.

Overcoming Common Problems Series

For a full list of titles please contact
Sheldon Press, Marylebone Road, London NW1 4DU

Overcoming Common Problems Series

Overcoming Common Problems Series

Overcoming Common Problems

Coping with
Rheumatism and Arthritis

Dr Robert M. Youngson

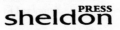

First published in Great Britain in 1998 by
Sheldon Press, SPCK, Marylebone Road, London NW1 4DU

© Dr Robert M. Youngson 1998

British Library Cataloguing-in-Publication Data
A catalogue record for this book is available from the British Library

ISBN 0–85969–785–1

Photoset by Deltatype Limited, Birkenhead, Merseyside
Printed in Great Britain by
Biddles Ltd, Guildford and King's Lynn

Contents

No medical book written for non-medical people, however much useful detail it may contain, can ever replace a consultation with a qualified doctor. During a consultation, you are being observed, questioned and examined by the doctor, and the direction the consultation takes will be affected by what the doctor hears and sees. Although there is much in this book that may be of the greatest importance to you, it is not intended to replace your doctor or to discourage you from seeking professional medical advice.

If anything in the book suggests to you that you are suffering from any of the major conditions with which it deals, you are urged to see your doctor without delay. The author has made every effort to ensure that the contents of this book reflect up-to-date orthodox medical opinion, but no book of this kind can claim to contain the last word on any medical matter.

Introduction

After cancer and heart disease, arthritis is the most common health problem in Britain and Europe. More than 20 million people in Britain have at least one episode of arthritis each year. Five million of them have some degree of osteoarthritis and about half a million have rheumatoid arthritis. The rheumatic diseases constitute a substantial proportion of the workload of doctors – about 1 in 5 of all medical consultations are for this range of disorders. Even more serious, rheumatic diseases are responsible for 30 per cent of all physical disability. In the case of older people, some 60 per cent of their total severe disability is caused by these disorders. The amount of suffering, especially among those with established long-term arthritis, is enormous. Lost working time from arthritic disorders may also involve major financial hardship.

It is therefore important for you to know as much as possible about the rheumatic diseases so that you can seek early treatment and, so far as is possible, limit the advancement of any joint problem you may have. This book is written in simple, direct language, avoiding technical expressions, with the aim of providing you with exactly the knowledge you need. By reading it you will be able to decide whether your problems are minor or whether they are potentially serious. You should be able to identify what form of rheumatic disorder you have, and then read about the very latest treatments available.

This is not, of course, a do-it-yourself arthritis management handbook. It would be dangerous to try to handle this kind of problem on your own. But the more you know about the subject, the more effectively will you be able to ensure you get the best treatment.

1

All about joints

Joints are places where bones come together and are linked in various ways. Many junctions between bones allow fairly free movement, but some do not. There are three kinds of joints – fibrous, cartilaginous, and synovial. Don't worry about these names – they will be explained in a moment. Fibrous joints, such as those between the bones of the top of the skull, allow little or no movement; the bones concerned are bound firmly together. Cartilaginous joints, such as those between the ribs and the breast-bone or between the bodies of the bones of the spine, allow some rather limited stiff bending movement. In this case, the bones are joined by a piece of gristle.

Synovial joints are the kind this book is concerned with. They are the kind of joints you have at your shoulder, elbow, hip and knee, and are enclosed in capsules and reinforced by internal and external ligaments. They are freely movable joints, and have lubricated bearing surfaces. Because they are constantly rubbing against one another, these bearing surfaces need to be hard-wearing. To provide suitable surfaces, the articular ends of the bones are covered with a special kind of cartilage which, when suitably lubricated, provides a smooth gliding surface offering very low levels of friction. This is called the articular cartilage. The lubricating fluid, or synovial fluid, comes from a layer on the inner surface of the joint capsule called the synovial membrane.

The synovial membrane

The inner surface of the joint capsule is well provided with blood vessels and active cells so that it can constantly secrete a lubricating fluid – synovial fluid. This is a colourless to deep yellow fluid that, although 95 per cent water, is quite viscous and slightly sticky – about the same as the white of an egg, hence the name ('synovia' means 'like an egg'). The viscosity of synovial fluid varies with temperature – a fact that may account for winter joint stiffness. As a lubricant, in conjunction with articular cartilage, synovial fluid is highly efficient, achieving a level of friction lower than that of ice sliding on ice. Some absorption of synovial fluid occurs into the articular cartilages, and when joints are subjected to high pressures this fluid is squeezed out, thereby providing the extra lubrication required under these circumstances.

The joint cartilage

The cartilage covering the bearing surfaces of the bones, the articular cartilage, contains no blood vessels, and gets its nourishment – oxygen, sugar, minerals and so on – mainly from the synovial fluid that lubricates it. This nutritional supply allows the cartilage to renew itself over the years, to make up for wear and tear. Barring accidents or excessive stresses, such as from excess weight or disease, articular cartilage should continue to function normally throughout life.

The articular cartilage is firmly bound to the ends of the bones. But some joints, such as the knee, have additional cartilages that assist in the mechanics of the joint and are less firmly attached. These are called articular discs – tough inserts reinforced with fibrous tissue and connected to the joint capsule at their edges. They act as shock absorbers and as pressure sensors, sending information to the brain about pressure changes within the joint. In order to do this, they are provided with nerves.

Joint capsules and ligaments

Joints are enclosed in tough, fibrous capsules. Each capsule consists of a number of very strong bands of fibres forming virtual ligaments that are incorporated into a continuous, less dense sheet of fibre. These capsular ligaments play an important part in holding the bones together in the proper relationship, but they are not the only structures performing this function. One or more powerful ligamentous cords run directly from one bone to the other, actually within the joint. These internal ligaments also have an important function in limiting the joint movement to certain directions and restricting the range of movement. They are usually in a state of tension when the joint is in its most stable position. Muscles and muscle tendons, which operate across joints, also play an important part in maintaining joint stability, as does the actual shape of the bearing surfaces.

Ligaments have much in common with tendons, and differ mainly in shape. They are strong, flexible bands attached to bone, usually acting to bind bones together, either tightly or loosely. Bones often provide special prominences, called processes, to which ligaments are attached. Ligaments are formed from tightly parallel bundles of collagen, have a shiny white appearance, and are pliable and flexible. Their attachment to bone is so secure that sometimes bone will fracture rather than allow ligaments to tear off. Most ligaments are relatively non-elastic, but some are formed from yellow elastic fibres and are able to stretch enough to allow connected bones to separate slightly.

There are more kinds of joints than you probably realize. Note that while the actual shape of the joint surfaces determines to a large extent the degree of freedom of movement, this is always further limited by the capsular and other ligaments associated with the joint. Here are some details of the different types of joints in the body.

Types of joint

Hinge joints

These allow movement in one plane only. An example is the joint at the elbow between the upper arm bone (humerus) and the inner of the two bones of the forearm (ulna). In this joint, a curved convex surface fits into, and rotates within, a curved concave surface.

Ball and socket joints

These allow exceptional freedom of movement in all directions. An example is the hip joint, in which the almost spherical head of the thigh bone (femur) sockets into the deep hemispherical cavity on the side of the pelvis – the acetabulum (a word derived from the Latin word for a vinegar cup). The shoulder joint is another ball and socket joint.

Pivot joints

These allow rotation only. An example is the joint between the upper two neck bones (vertebrae), the atlas and the axis. Some joints, such as the one between the upper end of the outer forearm bone (radius) and the lower end of the humerus, allow a hinge movement as well as pivoting.

Ellipsoidal joints

In this type of joint, an elliptical or egg-shaped bulge fits into a cavity of similar shape. This allows motion in two planes at right angles to each other, but limits rotation. An example of an ellipsoidal joint is the one between the lower end of the forearm radius bone and the scaphoid bone of the wrist group.

Gliding joints

In gliding joints, the surfaces are almost flat or slightly convex and concave, but the bones are secured by ligaments so that any rotation is prevented. An example is the joint between adjacent articular surfaces on the arches of the vertebrae of the spine.

Fixed and almost fixed joints

Fixed joints allow no movement. Examples are the 'sutures' between the bones of the top of the skull. These complicated 'jig-saw' joints are readily visible on the vault of the cranium. The bones are joined by a thin layer of fibrous tissue, but the nature of the junction makes separation almost impossible. We will not be concerned with this kind of joint. Slightly movable joints, however, are important in the context of rheumatism and arthritis. In these, the bones may be fixed together by short, dense ligaments, as in the case of the sacro-iliac joints between the sides of the central rear bone of the pelvis – the sacrum – and the outer bones of the pelvis. Slightly movable joints may also be secured by a pad of fibrous cartilage, as in the case of the midline front joint between the two side pubic parts of the pelvic bones. This joint is called the symphysis pubis (a symphysis is just a firm junction between two parts).

Facts about joints

- The bearing (articular) surface of joints is a layer of cartilage with a beautiful, pearly, silvery-blue polished lustre. Its surface cells are arranged in parallel rows. It has no nerves and damage produces no pain. When worn away, however, the underlying sensitive bone may be exposed, which can result in pain.
- The inner lining membrane of joints, the synovial membrane, as well as lining the joint capsule, also encloses and covers all internal ligaments and plates of fibrocartilage (cartilage strengthened by protein (collagen) fibres), keeping them from contact with the synovial fluid.
- In many joints, the limitation of movement between the bones is achieved exclusively by ligaments.
- Some healthy people have a wider range of joint movement than average. This may be inborn or may be due to activities

---

such as Hatha Yoga. Most people with an unusual range of movement in a joint, however, are suffering from injury to a ligament or from a joint malformation or disease. In some cases they may be suffering from an inherited disorder of connective tissue in which the collagen structure is abnormal, allowing undue laxity of ligaments. The main forms of this disorder are called the Ehlers–Danlos syndrome and Marfan's syndrome. Most common joint diseases cause *limitation* of movement.

- The joints between the bones of the pelvis, although normally almost immovable, become more lax during pregnancy so as to ease the passage of the baby's head. This change is largely due to the increased blood flow in the area.

2

What are the rheumatic disorders?

Rheumatism is a general term for the wide range of conditions that cause pain in or around one or more joints, resulting in stiffness and varying degrees of disablement. The term arthritis is rather more specific, but still refers to a considerable number of different conditions. Strictly speaking, arthritis means 'inflammation in a joint' – the word-ending *-itis* means 'inflammation of'. But with advances in medical knowledge it has become clear that at least one of the important conditions long described as an arthritis – osteoarthritis – does not actually involve inflammation. The name, however, is now so firmly established that it is hard to change.

Many medical conditions whose names have traditionally ended in -itis are now better understood and are being renamed, usually with *-opathy* as an ending. Medical purists are keen to replace the general term arthritis with the term arthropathy, but as this may take some time, we will stick with arthritis for present purposes. The majority of arthritides (plural of arthritis) actually do involve inflammation.

Arthritis covers conditions that actually affect joints, but these, of course, commonly also involve the soft tissues around the joints. Some of the arthritides are not simply confined to the joints but have widespread effects throughout the body – rheumatoid arthritis is a case in point. Some have strong associations with disorders in quite remote parts of the body – it is, for instance, quite common for people with certain rheumatic disorders to develop potentially serious inflammation inside one or both eyes. This is important information that can be sight-saving for the people concerned.

Many of the conditions have other important complications and, in many cases, the most effective treatments available themselves involve a degree of risk. It is not widely understood that rheumatic disorders are often the result of general disease. A disorder such as Lyme arthritis, for example, can be avoided altogether if the early symptoms of the disease are recognized, enabling the condition to be treated. Some forms of arthritis – such as septic arthritis – call for very urgent treatment if a serious outcome is to be avoided – indeed, it is partly to help avoid such outcomes that this book has been written.

The range of rheumatic disorders

There are about 200 different kinds of rheumatic disease, most of which are rare and seldom seen, but some of which are common. Subsequent chapters cover all the common and some of the more frequently encountered rare kinds, dealing with such conditions as osteoarthritis (osteoarthropathy), rheumatoid arthritis, tennis elbow and frozen shoulder, gout, ankylosing spondylitis, cervical spondylosis, repetitive strain injury, carpal tunnel syndrome, rotator cuff syndrome, bursitis, polymyalgia rheumatica, systemic lupus erythematosus, Lyme disease and rheumatic fever (all these strange-sounding terms will be fully explained).

Oddly enough, the rheumatic disorders do not affect the sexes equally. While several of them are far commoner in women than in men, a few are commoner in men. It is not at all clear why this should be. Certainly the reason has nothing to do with the fact that some men engage in more traumatic work than women, for the joints and the surrounding soft tissue actually thrive on heavy usage. The one thing that is really bad for them is disuse – a joint prevented from moving for a year will go almost solid, and is unlikely ever to recover its full range of movement.

A few of the rheumatic disorders occur only in childhood. Others start in early adult life, while many rarely appear before the middle 50s.

Importance of duration

One of the main features distinguishing serious or potentially serious rheumatic conditions from trivial conditions is the length of time they have been present. Few if any people go through life without suffering at least a few episodes of rheumatic pain and stiffness. In many cases such episodes follow immediately on an injury or an unusual bout of exertion or injudicious deliberate exercising. They may also follow a period of enforced immobilization due to another illness. In all such cases, the cause of the symptoms is obvious, the duration of the problem is brief and, unless the injury, say, was severe, full recovery is to be expected.

Conditions that come on gradually or insidiously, with progressive worsening and long duration, are in quite a different category. These are likely to be what are called 'chronic' conditions, and they are likely to cause trouble. Note that the word chronic says nothing about the severity of the disorder (it comes from the Greek word *chronos*, meaning 'time', and simply means long-lasting). Unfortunately, chronic conditions may last for a life-time. Because of this, they are necessarily more serious than acute conditions, which although often sharper and more severe, last for only a short time.

However, while in the past most chronic conditions, whether mild or severe, were a life-sentence, today, happily, some can be entirely cured by modern methods of treatment (such as joint replacement surgery), and many others so well controlled by medication that quality of life is little affected.

Long-term effects on the body

Many chronic rheumatic conditions are mild and bring about little or no visible changes in the body. Some, of course, do result in walking and other visible movement difficulties – slowing, limping, postural changes and the need to use walking or other aids can make the more severe chronic conditions conspicuous. The most obvious bodily changes occur in conditions, such as rheumatoid arthritis and ankylosing spondylitis, that can produce widespread structural changes.

These things are mentioned to make the point that the best medical and surgical management of rheumatic disorders is not directed simply at the relief of pain and disability. The aim of treatment must always be to reduce to the absolute minimum the *appearance* of disorder, so that physical suffering is not compounded by feelings of possible social disadvantage.

One of the commonest ways in which rheumatic disorders can affect appearance is by bringing about severe limitation of joint movement. This can affect both bodily posture and the normality of movement. A few years ago, I was hit by a car and sustained a serious compound thigh bone fracture. This refused to heal, and for several months my leg was totally immobilized. The result was a knee that would not bend. When the bone was finally fixed with an internal steel rod, the worst feature of the condition was a fixed knee. A well-meaning physiotherapist informed me that the fixation of the joint was permanent, and showed me some professional papers to prove it!

Happily, I had other ideas, and decided to prove the physiotherapist wrong and to work on the knee on my own. It took about six months, but by constant effort to bend the knee, the range of flexion very slowly and gradually increased. Today the movement is full and, in appearance and function, my knee is entirely normal.

9

Occupation and the rheumatic disorders

The whole of the skeletal system – bones, joints, muscles, tendons and ligaments – may be affected by particular occupations. Bones may suffer weakening (osteoporosis) from sedentary occupation, or hair-line fractures from repetitive force; joints may be overloaded and suffer progressive arthritic changes; muscles may be fatigued, cramped or inflamed; ligaments may be stretched or torn; and tendons and their sheaths inflamed and stiffened in their action by overuse.

One of the principal occupational causes of rheumatic disorder is repetitive heavy impact on bones, joints and soft tissues around joints. This is the reason why, in the past, so many men engaged in manual labour – in mines and quarries, on roads, in civil engineering generally and in agriculture and other trades – so often ended up with severe joint problems from osteoarthritis (see Chapter 4). The constantly repeated trauma to these parts led to severe degenerative changes in joints, and to swelling and inflammation in the overlying tissues. To some extent, joints are protected from such trauma by small fibrous bags of fluid called bursas. These react to excess impact by thickening, becoming inflamed and secreting excess fluid – a condition known as bursitis (see Chapter 8). Occupations once particularly likely to produce bursitis were those involving much work while kneeling – 'housemaid's knee' was a case in point.

Repetitive low-impact stresses to certain parts, especially the hands, also give rise to rheumatic problems affecting the fingers, wrists and forearms. This has become much commoner in the last 20 years or so, and is widely attributed to the enormous increase in the use of computer keyboards. The subject is complicated, and all kinds of psychological, as well as physical, factors are involved. The term 'repetitive strain injury' (see Chapter 8) has been widely used to refer to distressing effects arising in this way. There is little doubt that lack of attention in the past to the physical relationship of the person to the work environment (ergonomics) has led to many people suffering unnecessary rheumatic damage. Happily, this situation is rapidly being corrected.

3

How rheumatic disorders are diagnosed

This chapter is primarily concerned with how doctors go about deciding exactly what kind of rheumatic disorder, if any, is present. But there is much in it that will help you decide for yourself what kind of trouble you may have, and whether it is likely to be minor or potentially serious. Do remember, however, the warning given at the beginning of this book. Diagnosis is a job for a doctor, and the diagnosis, or the failure to make a correct diagnosis, may have important consequences for you.

Because the most important joints, from the point of view of mobility and freedom, are the hip and knee joints, it is on the diagnosis of problems with these joints that this chapter will concentrate. Much of the detail, however, applies to other joints.

The history

The most important part of any medical consultation is the taking of the history – the careful questioning of the patient about anything that has happened to him or her in the past that could have a bearing, however indirectly, on the present medical condition. A doctor concerned with a rheumatic or arthritic condition will be interested in quite a number of points. These will include such things as:

- family history of any rheumatic disorder;
- other serious illnesses;
- previous injuries;
- history of the present complaint;
- when it started;
- where the pain is;
- how severe it is;
- its characteristics;
- whether intermittent or permanent;
- what brings it on;
- what makes it worse;
- how much disability it causes;
- what other symptoms are associated with it.

The site of the pain may be misleading. This is especially so with hip arthritis. In addition, pain may be thought to arise in the hip when, in fact, it does not: people with pain in the buttock will often attribute this to a hip problem when it may actually be due to a slipped disc; pain originating in the abdomen – perhaps from a kidney stone, a hernia, a swelling (aneurysm) in the main artery, or an infection – may be wrongly attributed to a hip problem; pain assumed to be of rheumatic origin may actually be due to secondary cancer. In fact pain originating in the hip joint is felt on the front of the thigh or deep in the groin. It may be absent at rest, start as soon as the sufferer begins to walk or even to stand up. It often gets worse as walking or weight bearing continues. With very severe hip problems, the pain may be present even at rest, and may seriously disturb sleep.

Physical examination of the hip

In degenerative hip disorders such as osteoarthritis, there is often progressive loss of freedom to move about. To begin with, it may not be noticed. Eventually, however, the affected person begins to realize that he or she is finding it increasingly difficult to put on their shoes, dress, get in and out of the car, and so on. Climbing stairs may get much harder, and the person will come to rely more and more on the banisters. Walking becomes slower, and the distance it is possible to walk decreases.

Pain in the hip leads to a method of walking that is consciously or unconsciously calculated to minimize the pain. Because bearing weight on the affected side hurts, the gait is adjusted to minimize the time weight is borne on that side. Often the joint will not extend fully, and a stiff joint may make it impossible to put the leg flat when lying flat on one's back. All these things will be checked by the doctor, who will pay particular attention to the gait. To the trained eye, this can indicate not only the probable site and nature of the problem, but also the severity and degree of disability.

By direct physical examination, the doctor will assess the amount of stiffness present and the range of motion in the joint concerned. He or she will also wish to check whether there is any shortening in the muscles that bend (flex) the hip. This can be done with a simple test in which both knees are brought up towards the chest, and then the leg on the unaffected side is held there while the other leg is allowed to straighten as far as possible. If extension is incomplete, the muscles

12

have shortened. This is called a flexion contracture and, ideally, it should be prevented from happening.

The doctor will then test the freedom with which the whole leg can be rotated inwards. This movement can occur only at the hip joint, so is an important indication of the state of the joint. If internal rotation causes pain, it is often an indication of early hip degeneration. As the condition worsens, it may become impossible for the leg to rotate internally. Severe hip joint problems, such as collapse of the spherical head of the thigh bone due to loss of its blood supply, will cause an apparent or real shortening of the leg. Comparison of leg length is therefore an important part of the examination – measurements are taken on both sides from corresponding bony points on the pelvis to the bony bump on the inside of the ankle, and from the navel to the ankle bone.

The examination will also include an assessment of the strength of the muscles that move the joint. This is done on both sides, so that comparisons can be made. In the case of the hip joint, because of its wide range of movements, there are more of these muscles than you might imagine.

X-ray is another important part of the examination. In the case of osteoarthritis of the hip joint, one of the most striking changes to be seen on X-ray is the loss of the normal space between the ball at the head of the hip bone (femur) and the cup into which it fits. This space is readily visible all round the head in a healthy hip joint, but becomes strikingly narrowed as the disease progresses. The narrowing is first noted between the upper part of the ball and the cup, where the greatest force is applied when bearing weight. Joint space narrowing is an important X-ray finding in all cases of arthritis. It is an indication that articular cartilage has been at least partially destroyed. Cartilage is much less dense to X-ray than bone, and does not show up well – the space seen on X-ray is really the space occupied by the cartilage rather than an actual space.

Other X-ray signs include increased density in the bone around the joint, and the presence of abnormal bony outgrowths, called osteo-phytes, on the edges of the joint. In severe cases, the actual partial destruction of the head of the femur can be seen.

Computer tomography (CT scanning) and magnetic resonance imagining (MRI) are also often used to examine joints. The former provides the most detailed information on subtle changes in the bones, while the latter provides most detail on soft tissue changes. Other special methods of examination include the removal of a little of the joint fluid by needle and syringe for examination, and the use of fine optical instruments that are passed into the joint for direct inspection. This is called arthroscopy and is becoming widely used, not only for direct inspection but also to allow delicate surgery to be performed under direct vision within the joint.

Physical examination of the knee

Again, the clinical history is of the greatest importance. The doctor will be especially interested in a history of knee injury of any kind, as this often gives rise to later trouble. A history of fractures of the adjacent parts of the bones forming the knee joint – the lower thigh bone, the upper lower leg bone and the kneecap (patella) – is also important. Injury to the cartilages of the knee or to any of the internal or external ligaments must also be known. The doctor is especially interested in a history of the knee giving way, or locking, and of episodes of swelling.

Surprisingly, pain in the knee may not necessarily indicate any knee problem. Such pain can be referred from a diseased hip joint or even from the lower spine. In this case, the further examination of the knee may reveal no organic abnormality. Many different conditions can cause knee pain, and doctors recognize that it is important not simply to assume that the condition is osteoarthritis. A painful or swollen knee may be the result of injury, but it may also be caused by internal infection, rheumatoid arthritis, gout, pseudo-gout or other disorders.

Examination of the knee begins with visual inspection and observation of how the affected person stands and walks. An important point is to compare the two knees – any obvious difference, such as in the degree of warmth, is noted. Swelling or enlargement may be due to a collection of fluid in the joint, known as effusion, or to thickening of the capsule. These causes can be easily distinguished. Fluid can be made to move by sudden squeezing, alternately above and below the kneecap (patella). It can also be detected by pressing the patella sharply back, when it will be felt to bounce on the lower end of the thigh bone (the patellar tap test).

With the person being examined sitting, the foot on the ground, and the knee at right angles, the lower leg can be pushed back and pulled forward. If movement is possible there is laxity of the internal ligaments. With the person lying and the legs perfectly straight, an attempt is then made to see if any sideways movement, inwards or outwards, is possible at the knee. No such movement should occur. If it does, the indication is that there is weakness of the outer (collateral) ligaments on either side of the knee.

Arthritis will usually result in at least some limitation of bending and straightening (flexion and extension) of the joint. Defective alignment and a tendency to swing the leg outward when walking are subtle indications of the presence of joint disease.

The active and passive range of motion are noted at the time of examination. Side-to-side movement of the kneecap with moderate backward pressure may produce a grinding sensation suggesting some disease of the articular cartilage on the back of the bone.

X-ray examination of the knee from front to back and side to side, and sometimes in other directions, can provide much useful information. It can show:

- fluid in the joint;
- narrowing of the joint space;
- increase in bone density (sclerosis);
- irregular bony outgrowths from the margins (osteophytes);
- deformity in the joint;
- cysts under the bearing cartilages;
- loose pieces of cartilage (loose bodies);
- actual loss of bone.

Doctors will always arrange for X-rays suggestive of early joint disease to be preserved. Comparisons of X-rays over a period provides invaluable information on the progress or otherwise of a disease process. In most people with rheumatic disorders of fairly short duration, the X-ray appearances are unlikely to be abnormal. In rheumatoid arthritis, changes in the X-ray, such as joint space narrowing or damage to the joint margins, are unlikely to be visible until at least six months have passed. People with osteoarthritis, however, will show X-ray indication of joint damage. This is because in osteoarthritis symptoms that draw the attention of the person to the problem do not occur until significant damage has already been done. Magnetic resonance imaging (MRI) is very useful for showing up disease of soft tissue in and around the affected joint, and is being increasingly used. It provides more detailed information than straight X-rays.

A sample of fluid in the knee joint is commonly obtained by sucking it out through a needle (aspiration) with a syringe. This is especially important if there is any question of infection. When people have symptoms of sudden onset in only one joint, with joint swelling and a raised joint temperature, it is necessary to assume that the trouble is septic arthritis until proved otherwise. Septic arthritis is extremely damaging, and it must be treated as soon as possible with the correct antibiotic (aspiration allows the organisms to be identified).

Direct visual inspection of the inside of the joint (arthroscopy) is now widely practised and, for many surgeons, is the preferred method of confirming the diagnosis, planning treatment, recording progress and carrying out various operative procedures. It is not, however, considered a substitute for the methods of history-taking and physical examination described. Arthroscopy can provide unique information about the inside of a joint, but, as always, medicine is concerned with the whole individual, not just one small part.

4

Arthritis without inflammation – osteoarthritis

It is worth repeating that the term osteoarthritis is misleading. The word ending -itis means 'inflammation', and although in the late stages of severe cases some of the soft tissues may become inflamed, the basic features of the disease do not include inflammation. The name, however, is so well established that to use the more accurate term osteoarthropathy would probably cause confusion.

Osteoarthritis is the commonest of all forms of established arthritic disease, and is believed to be present, to some degree, in the weight-bearing joints, especially the knees, in nearly everyone over the age of about 40. Ten to fifteen per cent of people over 45 suffer pain and disability from osteoarthritis of the knee. In Britain alone, more than two million adults have osteoarthritis of the knee, or knees, of sufficient severity to cause pain and disability. The disease affects the sexes about equally, but tends to show itself earlier in men than in women. Interestingly, the trouble is not confined to humans – it is common in all large animals. The characteristic changes can even be found in the remains of dinosaurs.

Causes of osteoarthritis

Until recently, no one really had any idea of why osteoarthritis occurs. Most doctors assumed that it was simply a 'wearing out' disease in which the bearing surfaces of the weight-bearing joints became damaged by constant use. This idea was supported by the observation that the condition tends to be worse in people who are overweight. General environmental factors, such as occupation, have also been thought to be important, but to date there has been no conclusive evidence to support this view.

Recent research at St Thomas' Hospital, London, reported in the British Medical Journal in 1996, suggests, for the first time, that there is a hereditary basis for osteoarthritis. This careful study, carried out on 130 identical twins and 120 non-identical twins, recorded the presence or absence of osteoarthritic changes and other features of the disease in the knees and hands of all those studied. When the data were analysed, it was found that in a high proportion of the identical twins, when one had obvious osteoarthritis, the other also had it to a similar degree. In the case of the non-identical twins, the correlation between the pairs was much lower.

Identical twins have exactly the same genes. Non-identical twins share, on average, half their genes. Thus, if identical twins have differences, these differences must be due not to genetics but to environmental factors. In the case of non-identical twins, differences may be due to both genetic and environmental factors. The fact that the identical twins were found to be so similar in respect to osteoarthritis strongly implies, without actually proving, that genetic factors are important in this disease. The predisposition to osteoarthritis does not absolutely ensure that the disease will occur, but it does make it much more likely. Future research is likely to prove that both heredity and environment are important in causing osteoarthritis.

A number of other factors are known to be important. Almost any disease that can in any way change the cartilage-bearing surface of the joints can lead to osteoarthritis. These include:

- mechanical injury;
- excessive pressure from weight;
- change in the physical relationship of the bone ends, as from rickets, bow-legs, knock-knees, congenital deformities etc.;
- overuse of certain joints;
- infection;
- damage to the joint nerve supply;
- hormonal disorders;
- other joint diseases, such as gout or rheumatoid arthritis.

Although many forms of work trauma are known to cause osteoarthritis, certain forms of overuse do not. The reason for this is obscure. In spite of the constant and long-continued pounding, workers with pneumatic drills do not get more osteoarthritis of the arm or hand joints; and long-distance runners do not get more osteoarthritis of the knees or other leg joints.

Osteoarthritis that has obvious environmental or disease causes is called secondary osteoarthritis. Osteoarthritis with no such obvious causes is known as primary osteoarthritis. Primary osteoarthritis can affect almost any joint, including those of the hands, feet, spine, knee and hip.

How joints are affected

We have seen that healthy joints in healthy bodies do not suffer wear. The excellent lubrication system of the synovial membrane and fluid ensures this. 'Dirty oil' is automatically removed from the joint into the joint veins and carried away. New lubricant is then secreted by the synovial membrane. Very small particles of debris are also removed from the joint. Even if some physical damage does occur, scattered cells in the cartilage called chondrocytes can generate new cartilage to make up deficits. These cells are very quiet and dormant, and start working only if damage has occurred.

When things start to go wrong – for whatever reason – there is an increased production of new bone in the surface under the bearing cartilage, and some abnormal increase in the production of cartilage. As new bone forms, the bone under the cartilage loses its elasticity and numerous tiny fractures occur in it. This starts up a vicious cycle of more stiffness and more fractures. Sooner or later, bony protrusions (osteophytes) develop at the edges of the joint. These are readily visible on X-ray, as we have seen.

Next, the bearing cartilage and the underlying bone develop faults or clefts, so that synovial fluid is forced right through into the marrow of the bone. This causes visible marrow cysts and a scarring and bone-production reaction around these abnormal sites. The result is obvious roughening, irregularity and pitting, and then actual patchy loss of the articular cartilage surface. As well as new bone formation, there is a further attempt to repair the damage in the form of increased growth of joint tendons, synovial membrane and joint capsule – in fact, of all the structure of the joint. At this final stage in the process, osteoarthritis may show an inflammatory element in the synovial membrane. Inflammation does not affect the joint cartilage or the bone – since the cartilage has no blood vessels, it is incapable of developing inflammation.

Symptoms

The onset of osteoarthritis is gradual, and symptoms usually begin in one, or one or two, joints. The first indication is pain, which is usually worse on using the joint. After resting, stiffness is common but, to begin with, this generally lasts only for about 15 to 30 minutes and soon disappears as one gets moving. As the condition gradually gets worse, there is progressive reduction in the range through which the affected joints can be moved. If the disorder is neglected, the result of this progressive reduction is tightening and shortening of the muscles that normally move the joint. This in turn results in permanent inability to straighten the joint fully – a state known as a flexion contracture (see page 13).

Now the sufferer begins to be aware of a grating sensation on moving the joint, and there may even be tenderness on pressure to the joint. In the later stage of the process, there is joint enlargement resulting from increased growth of bone, cartilage, ligament, tendon, synovial membrane and joint capsule. As noted above, inflammation may now occur – which, of course, adds to the pain.

In the case of the knee, tendon overgrowth can cause instability in the joint, which may dislocate. An initial limitation of joint movement may therefore sometimes be followed by an abnormally wide range of movement. (Dislocation of the hip from osteoarthritis is uncommon, but limitation and pain may be severe.) Sometimes a knee joint will lock because pieces of bone or cartilage have come loose and are jammed inside. Osteophytes can also lock a joint. At this stage, there is a tendency for the muscles surrounding the joint to go into spasm. This, too, makes the pain worse.

In the case of osteoarthritis of the spine – which is quite common – the bone overgrowth can cause compression of the spinal cord that runs down through a series of holes in the separate bones of the spine (vertebrae). This compression can cause severe symptoms, including numbness and weakness. In the neck, two important arteries, the vertebral arteries, run up through a separate series of holes in the side processes of the bones. These arteries may also be compressed by osteophyte formation.

Osteoarthritis of the hands features appearances known as Heberden's nodes. These are unsightly bony excrescences (exostoses) the size of a small pea, occurring on the terminal bones of the fingers. They are really osteophytes in the form of enlargements of the normal bony bumps, or tubercles, at the edges of the outer joint, and are quite characteristic of osteoarthritis. Although the pain in the hands associated with Heberden's nodes will always settle, the nodes remain. William Heberden (1710–1801) was an English physician who made a name for himself by noticing and recording things like this.

Outlook

Osteoarthritis is very variable in its progression, but without treatment, the general tendency is to progressive worsening. This is not, however, invariable, and some cases actually get better spontaneously. Because the changes occur long before symptoms first appear, there is no practical way of trying to change the outcome at the earliest stages. From the onset of symptoms, however, management should be energetic, so as to limit both progress of the disease and erosion of quality of life. It is important to appreciate, however, that for most people the presence of osteoarthritis does not mean severe disability in later life. For most of us, the level of symptoms and the amount of disablement can readily be tolerated.

Treatment

There are several aspects to treatment, including:

- prevention of worsening;
- maximal rehabilitation of existing osteoarthritic problems;
- measures to limit worsening;
- control of pain;
- adjustment of lifestyle;
- maintenance of maximal fitness.

Treatment thus involves a clear understanding of the condition and of the factors that make it worse. People with osteoarthritis who are willing to co-operate with their doctors in its management can usually expect excellent results.

The first step is to shed excess weight. This, in itself, can greatly reduce the severity of symptoms. At the same time, an exercise programme must be set up that is designed to improve general health and the health of affected joints, and, by regular stretching, to increase their range of movement. These exercises, which will also strengthen muscles and tendons, improve posture and maintain healthy joint cartilages, are most important, and should be performed daily. They must be prescribed by your doctor and persisted with under medical or paramedical supervision – physiotherapists are trained in this work.

This is a situation in which immobilization is dangerous – it can speed the progress and worsen the outlook of the disease. On the other hand, a properly conducted exercise programme can halt the progress and even, to some extent, reverse the severity of osteoarthritis of the hips and knees especially. To allow re-lubrication of bearing cartilages, exercising must be alternated with periods of daytime rest. Postural instruction is also important. You will be taught to avoid slumping into soft or reclining armchairs, and to sit properly in straight chairs. You will also be advised about how best to maintain your daily occupation, and about sleeping on a firm mattress.

Drugs

In osteoarthritis, drug treatment is of relatively minor importance compared with its use in conditions such as rheumatoid arthritis, and takes second place to the measures already mentioned. This is because inflammation is not an important part of the process, and infection is not involved. That leaves pain control and, in some cases, relief of muscle spasm. The humble aspirin, or one of the other non-steroidal anti-inflammatory drugs (NSAIDs), is often all that is required to relieve pain. Drugs occasionally used to relax muscle include diazepam (Valium, Diazemuls, Stesolid, Valclair, Diazepam Rectubes), carisoprodol (Carisoma), and methocarbamol (Robaxim, Robaxisal). It is very rarely necessary to resort to steroid drugs in osteoarthritis, but if you are interested in steroids, there is more about these drugs in the treatment section of the next chapter.

Joint replacement surgery (see Chapter 10) is considered only as a last resort, but should always be an option in very severe and disabling cases. The results are usually remarkably good.

For a general account of the treatment of rheumatic disorders, see Chapter 9.

5

Arthritis with inflammation – rheumatoid arthritis

Rheumatoid arthritis is more than arthritis; it is a general disease, often with quite widespread effects outside the joints. The most obvious indication, however, is the involvement of several joints, usually in a symmetrical manner, and the most obvious feature is inflammation. It is a very variable disease, with considerable changes in, and periods of relative freedom from, symptoms. Sometimes it is so mild as to barely recognizable, but it is often a more destructive disease than osteoarthritis.

Rheumatoid arthritis is two to three times more common in women than in men, and affects about one person in a hundred. It may start at any age, even in childhood, but most commonly appears between the ages of 26 and 50.

Causes of rheumatoid arthritis

Despite considerable research, the cause of rheumatoid arthritis remains unknown. There are, however, some clues. The disease is commoner in first-degree relatives of people with rheumatoid arthritis than in the general population. So to this extent, it can be said to run in families. If one identical twin develops rheumatoid arthritis, the other is also highly likely to develop it. Moreover, all people who have rheumatoid arthritis share a particular pattern of one of the chemical groups that determine tissue typing. Like blood groups, all body cells fall into one of a number of groups known as tissue types. The disease nearly always becomes less severe during pregnancy, and women who have been pregnant are less likely to develop rheumatoid arthritis than women who have not. The significance of this factor is not fully understood.

Many experts believe that a viral infection may be implicated in causation of the disease, and there is some evidence linking it with the virus that causes glandular fever. This virus is not thought actually to cause rheumatoid arthritis, but it is believed that the virus in some way causes the immune system to produce antibodies that attack the synovial membrane of the joints (see Chapter 1).

One extraordinary feature of the disease is that sufferers who then

23

develop AIDS experience an apparent complete recovery from their rheumatoid arthritis. This indicates that the helper T-cells are involved – it is the deficiency of these cells as a result of HIV damage that is the cause of AIDS. It has also been shown that a deliberate artificial attack on the helper T-cells will produce a marked, if short-lived, improvement in rheumatoid arthritis. Treatment with immunosuppressive drugs (see below) that produce an AIDS-like situation also greatly improves rheumatoid arthritis. Research has produced a considerable amount of information about the disease, much of it tantalizingly suggesting that a full explanation of the cause is just around the corner. So far, unfortunately, this has proved an illusion.

The nature of rheumatoid arthritis

A joint affected by rheumatoid arthritis shows certain characteristic features. The usually delicate synovial membrane becomes thickened, thrown into folds and covered with millions of inflammatory cells. Large number of pus cells also appear in the synovial fluid, and the volume of the fluid increases enormously (in health, it is present only to the extent of a thin lubricating film over the interior surfaces of the joint). The bearing cartilages of the joint, the internal ligaments and the inside of the joint capsule become covered with clotted blood serum (fibrin), into which many new blood vessels grow. Even scar tissue can develop. This inflammatory process, unless checked, leads to severe damage to the interior of the joint, with patchy loss of the bearing cartilage and weakening of other internal structures. The result is distortion and deformity.

Highly characteristic of rheumatoid arthritis are the rheumatoid nodules. These are seen in about one-third of people with the disease. They occur under the skin at sites subject to trauma, and consist of a mass of cells with a central core of dead tissue. They appear at the elbow and on the back of the forearm, and around tendons, especially those on the backs of the fingers and the Achilles tendon above the heel bone. They are firm, non-tender swellings varying greatly in size (from a few millimetres to several centimetres across).

Symptoms

These can come on quite suddenly, but in most cases the onset is gradual. Sometimes the trouble starts in more than one joint simultaneously, but it is more common for joints to be affected one after the other. Affected joints are sore to touch (tender), which is a highly characteristic feature of the disease.

Many different joints may be involved in rheumatoid arthritis. Those most commonly first affected are:

- joints between the finger bones;
- joints between the fingers and the palm bones (knuckle joints);
- joints between the toe bones and the foot bones;
- elbows;
- wrists;
- ankles.

Any joint can, however, be the first to be involved. Even the spine may be involved. Rheumatoid arthritis of the neck part of the vertebral column can lead to neurological complications.

A typical early symptom is stiffness. This is often worse on getting up in the morning, and usually lasts for at least half an hour. It will also occur after any period of prolonged inactivity. But stiffness is not, of course, specific to rheumatoid arthritis – it is involved in most forms of arthritis. Rheumatoid arthritis is a general disorder, producing general effects. It is, for instance, common for the affected person to feel sick and thoroughly fatigued in the early afternoon.

The most striking and, to many, distressing feature of rheumatoid arthritis is the deformity it causes. Affected joints tend to become partially fixed in a bent position. Characteristically, the fingers become deviated towards the side of the little finger, resulting in the tendons that run along the backs of the fingers, and that should tighten to straighten them, tending to slip sideways off the knuckle joints. The appearance is often made worse by rheumatoid nodules (see above).

Some of the general effects of rheumatoid arthritis may add to the general distress. They include:

- fever;
- loss of weight;
- recurrent infections;
- damage to small blood vessels;
- damage to nerves;
- leg ulcers;
- fluid in the pleural space around the lungs (pleural effusion);
- fluid in the bag surrounding the heart (pericardial effusion);
- enlarged lymph nodes;

- dry mouth (Sjögren's syndrome);
- dry eyes (Sjögren's syndrome);
- inflammation of the white of the eye (episcleritis).

Occasionally, the spleen is enlarged in long-term rheumatoid arthritis, which will draw attention particularly to the white cell count in the blood – a low white cell count in conjunction with an enlarged spleen and lymph nodes is called Felty's syndrome.

Diagnosis of rheumatoid arthritis

The clinical features just detailed, when fully developed, will usually be sufficient in themselves to make the diagnosis obvious. But it is usual to back up interpretation of the symptoms and signs with a number of laboratory tests, which usually reveal some additional features of the disease.

A routine blood test will, in a high proportion of cases, show that there is a significant degree of anaemia. Sometimes this is severe, calling for treatment in its own right – anaemia may be adding to the sufferer's problems, and its correction will always be beneficial. It may be partly due to iron deficiency (which is easy to treat), but anaemia wholly due to rheumatoid arthritis is difficult to treat while the disease is active, and does not respond to iron, vitamin B_{12} or folic acid. When the rheumatoid arthritis is controlled, however, the anaemia rapidly improves.

A laboratory indication of the severity of the rheumatoid arthritis is the red blood cell sedimentation rate (ESR). A sample of blood is drawn up in a graduated tube, which is set up vertically. After one hour, the distance to which the red cells have sedimented down is read off. This is not just a test for rheumatoid arthritis – an increased rate of sedimentation is caused by changes in the amount of a particular protein in the blood, and the test simply gives an indication of the general severity of a disease. It is, however, quite useful, and can even be critically important. In rheumatoid arthritis, the ESR is raised in 90 per cent of cases.

Perhaps the most important laboratory test for rheumatoid arthritis is the test for rheumatoid factors (these are antibodies produced by the immune system in response to altered gamma-globulin which is regarded as a 'foreign' substance. Again, although the finding of rheumatoid factors is not a 100 per cent positive indication of rheumatoid arthritis, it is highly suggestive. High levels of rheumatoid factors suggest severe disease, and the levels can drop if the condition is effectively treated.

In cases of doubt, it may be necessary to draw off a sample of synovial fluid for analysis. Analysis of the cellular and chemical content of the fluid can help to distinguish rheumatoid arthritis from other conditions. The internal appearance of the rheumatoid nodules is so highly characteristic that biopsy and microscopic examination can confirm the diagnosis.

Treatment

When rheumatoid arthritis is very active and causing considerable pain, a short period of complete bed rest may be prescribed. In cases of lesser severity, regular short periods of rest will be ordered. It is counter productive to keep people with rheumatoid arthritis in bed for long periods. Rest periods for badly affected joints are provided by splinting, which reduces joint inflammation and will often relieve pain. Up to three-quarters of people in their first year of rheumatoid arthritis improve with nothing more in the way of treatment than limited rest, splinting and the use of simple pain-killers.

It is most important to prevent the development of fixed bending of the joints (flexion contractures). This is done by gentle, passive straightening exercises, done carefully and within the limits of pain. When acute inflammation is controlled (see below), work can be done to maintain the strength of the muscles and retain the full range of joint movement. This will involve active rather than passive exercises. It must not, however, be pushed to the stage of causing fatigue. If flexion contractures have been allowed to become established, more intensive physiotherapy may be necessary.

Drug treatment is also important. The full benefits of exercise and physiotherapy cannot be obtained while the joints remain inflamed and painful. Here, surprisingly, one of the most useful drugs is aspirin. This is not just a pain-killer; it is also an effective anti-inflammatory medication. It is also fairly safe. Aspirin is usually started in a dosage of two to three tablets of 300 mg taken four times a day with food. The dosage is gradually increased until the effect is adequate or the drug starts to cause side effects, especially ringing in the ears (tinnitus) or deafness. High-dosage aspirin must be taken only under medical supervision – damage to the ears can be permanent, and the drug can cause considerable stomach irritation and even bleeding or ulceration in the stomach (special formulations that by-pass the stomach before being released are available). Some asthmatics are very sensitive to aspirin.

Other drugs in the same class as aspirin, non-steroidal anti-inflammatory drugs (NSAIDs), may be used by people who cannot tolerate enough aspirin or who prefer less frequent dosage. These include ibuprofen (Brufen, Codafen Continus, Motrin), indomethacin (Indocid, Indomod), fenoprofen (Fenopron, Progesic), naproxen (Naprosyn, Nycopren, Synflex), ketoprofen (Alrheumat, Ketocid, Orudis, Oruvail) and tolmetin (Tolectin). These drugs can also cause stomach irritation, and may induce asthma in allergic people. In some people they can cause headache or confusion, and they may raise blood pressure.

It is usual to try aspirin or other NSAIDs for a few months. If these do not sufficiently control the disease, more powerful drugs are required. A drug used increasingly to treat rheumatoid arthritis resistant to NSAIDs is sulphasalazine (Salazopyrin). Taken once a day by mouth in a gradually increasing dose, this usually produces a good response within about three months. The more powerful the drugs used, however, the more likely they are to have undesirable side effects, and this applies, unfortunately, to medication given for rheumatoid arthritis – sulphasalazine may cause headache, loss of appetite, nausea, skin rashes, damage to the blood-forming tissues, kidney damage and, in men, reduction in fertility.

The next step up in the hierarchy of treatments is into the major league, starting with gold. For many years, gold salts have been used successfully to treat rheumatoid arthritis. Gold can be highly effective, producing complete remission of the disease that can last for years. If, after a remission, the treatment is stopped for more than three to six months, the rheumatoid arthritis will usually recur, but by repeating the gold courses the benefit can often be continued indefinitely.

It is hardly necessary to mention that there are snags. Although often highly effective, gold salts can cause a number of adverse reactions. These include:

- stomach upset with diarrhoea, nausea and abdominal pain;
- disturbances of taste sensation;
- skin rashes;
- itching;
- loss of hair;

- damage to the blood;
- kidney damage;
- lung damage.

Anyone taking gold should be aware of the possibility of side effects, and should immediately report any new or unusual symptoms affecting any part of the body. The formulation most used in Britain is auranofin (Ridaura), a gold compound that can be taken by mouth. There are also gold preparations that can be given weekly by injection. Injected treatments do not produce nausea and other intestinal effects. Gold treatment is, of course, given only under close medical supervision.

There are dangers in giving gold preparations to people with liver or kidney disease, or to those with any disorder of the blood-forming tissues in the bone marrow. Blood and urine tests are necessary to check that all is well before starting gold treatment. In the event of severe reactions, metal-removing drugs can be used to get rid of the gold.

Another major drug, known as penicillamine (Distamine), which is derived from penicillin but is not an antibiotic, is capable of producing results similar to those of gold salts. It is often used in people who do not respond adequately to gold, or in whom the side effects of gold are too severe. Unfortunately, adverse effects with penicillamine are at least as common as with gold, and some of them can be even more serious: while in general the effects are similar, among a number of serious side effects penicillamine can cause is a form of severe weakness, amounting almost to partial paralysis, known as myasthenia gravis. There have been a few deaths from penicillamine, and the drug is used only by experts.

The third major drug used to control rheumatoid arthritis is hydroxychloroquine (Planequil). This is valuable in controlling moderately severe disease, and its side effects are, on the whole, mild. It is important that they should be known, however, and they include:

- skin inflammation (dermatitis);
- muscle disorders (myopathy);
- opacification of the corneas;
- retinal damage.

The last of these is the most important, and, once caused, the damage is permanent and irreversible. Because of this, people taking hydroxy-chloroquine must undergo regular examination by an eye specialist (ophthalmologist), including sensitive tests to check whether there is any damage to the peripheral fields of vision – we have no conscious awareness of patchy loss to the sides, and can even be tolerant, for a time, of the reduction in central visual sharpness. Careful and expert testing is thus required.

When the steroid drugs were first produced in the 1950s, it was thought that at last the ultimate treatment for rheumatoid arthritis had been found. The results in the initial stages of use were nothing short of miraculous. Symptoms were abolished, all the indications of inflammation disappeared and, in many cases, it looked as if the condition had been cured. Corticosteroids are the most powerful anti-inflammatory drugs available.

Regrettably, there are four major disadvantages that preclude the routine use of steroids. First, they do not cure rheumatoid arthritis and, with continued use, their effects usually diminish. Secondly, they do nothing to prevent the destructive changes in the joints. Thirdly, when they are stopped, the trouble recurs worse than ever (this is called the 'rebound phenomenon', and it can be serious). Finally, long-term use of steroids can have potentially dangerous side effects. These include:

- suppression of the body's own steroid production, leading to a dangerous collapse situation in the event of severe injury or surgery;
- danger of collapse on sudden withdrawal of drug;
- interference with the action of the immune system;
- reactivation of old infections;
- breakdown of healed wounds;
- production of bodily changes such as 'moon face';
- weight gain;
- acne;
- weakening of the bones (osteoporosis).

People on long-term steroids must carry a card or other indication for the use of doctors in an emergency. For all these reasons, after their initial enthusiasm, doctors have now abandoned the routine use of large-dose steroid treatment in rheumatoid arthritis. Steroids are still available, however, to cope with severe flare-ups and with some of the complications. In some cases, long-term, low-dosage steroids are deemed justified, and can be very effective. The dosage is strictly limited to about the same amount as is normally produced by the adrenal glands. Sometimes steroids are used by injection directly into severely affected joints. These powerful drugs are certainly effective, but as you can see, there are, unfortunately, major snags.

Since rheumatoid arthritis is known to be related to abnormal action of the immune system, there is now increasing use of drugs that suppress the action of the system. Immunosuppressive drugs, developed for use in transplant surgery to prevent rejection, are being increasingly used to control particularly severe rheumatoid arthritis. Drugs such as methotrexate and azathioprine can effectively reduce the severity of inflammation. Needless to say, the side effects are correspondingly severe. They are serious enough to limit the use of immunosuppressive drugs to the worst cases, and include such risks as liver damage, increased susceptibility to infection, interference with blood cell formation and an increased possibility of developing cancer. If your doctor is proposing to use them, you are entitled to a very full account of all the dangers. In general, they are prescribed only by specialists with experience in their use.

The question of whether people with rheumatoid arthritis should be treated *from the outset* with the range of powerful drugs described above has been widely raised in rheumatological circles. A recent review of this question, reported in the *British Medical Journal* in early 1997, provides support for early 'aggressive' treatment. A trial in the Netherlands suggested that people so treated are in significantly better shape after one year and after five years than people treated in the more conventional manner, described above, with non-steroidal anti-inflammatory drugs alone. However, because of the much higher level of side effects of these stronger drugs, and the need for close monitoring of people taking them, there is still considerable controversy on this point.

Much has been written in the popular medical press about the effect of diet on arthritis. This is a contentious subject, and a great deal of nonsense has been written. The experts are rightly suspicious of many of the claims, few of which are supported by properly conducted trials or real evidence. There are some reasonable suggestions that dietary supplements of various vegetable and fish oils may be helpful, but there is no more to it than that.

For a general account of the treatment of rheumatic disorders, see Chapter 9.

6

Crystals in the joints – gout

The image of the red-faced, port-swilling gouty colonel with his foot swathed in bandages has now, happily, been relegated to children's comics. Gout is not primarily caused by high living, although this does contribute to it, and a rich diet is now so common in the Western world that gout can no longer be considered the privilege of the upper classes. In fact, gout has become far more common than ever it was. In the United States the prevalence of gout has trebled in the last ten years – it is now the commonest cause of inflammatory arthritis in men over 40. Gout is also getting much more common in the UK. It primarily affects men, being about six times as common in men as in women. And it becomes commoner as age rises. Up to about the age of 40, the incidence in men is 2.4 per 1,000 of the population, but by the age of 60, this figure has risen to some 30 per 1,000. The younger the person is at the time the disease starts, the more severe it tends to be.

The nature of gout

Gout is an acute form of arthritis in which inflammation is caused by the deposition within the joint of crystals of a substance known as monosodium urate monohydrate. Any excess of uric acid in the body tends to lead to the formation of these crystals. Uric acid is relatively insoluble in water, and above a certain level the urate crystallizes out. Crystals are also deposited around the joints and tendons and in other tissues of the body, including the skin and the kidneys, where they may cause local damage. Sometimes the chalky crystals form nodules under the skin that can break through the skin (usually of the ear) to appear on the surface. These whitish, hard excrescences are called gouty tophi. It seems that the crystal deposits form more readily in skin that is exposed to the cold – hence the ears. About 15 per cent of people with gout also develop urate stones in their kidneys.

Crystal deposition occurs when the levels of uric acid in the blood (and in the body generally) rise much above the normal level. Uric acid is the end product of the breakdown in the liver of chemicals called purines, which are plentiful in the body because DNA is made, among other things, of purines. Purines are also fairly plentiful in the diet of most people. The amount of uric acid in the body depends on the balance of production of purines by the body, plus what is taken in the diet, and the rate at which uric acid is eliminated by the kidneys. A rise in the levels of uric acid may be the result of increased production of purines, decreased excretion of the kidneys, or both.

The commonest cause of a rise in the levels of uric acid, however, is a failure of the kidneys to excrete it fast enough. This is the cause of gout in at least 75 per cent of cases. The reason for this failure is still unclear, but it seems to be genetically determined – certainly, gout runs in families. Decreased excretion can also result from the use of diuretic drugs – drugs that increase the loss of water by the kidneys – and it also occurs if the kidneys have been damaged by disease.

In about 20 per cent of cases of gout, the cause is the other factor noted above, namely excessive production of uric acid as a result of increased production of purines. This is where high living does come in. After a meal of rich food there is a sharp rise in the levels of uric acid, especially if the meal has been washed down with a lot of wine. Alcohol has a dual effect in this respect: it causes the liver to break down purines more rapidly, and it interferes with the kidney's excretion of uric acid.

However, there is not a lot of point in ruining your life by living on a low-purine diet. This has only a very minor effect on the levels of uric acid in the body. If you are very diet conscious, however, you can bear in mind that purines are most present in foods that contain the highest concentrations of cells – foods like liver, sweetbreads (pancreas) and kidneys. Purine levels are also high in meats generally, so you can reduce your general animal protein intake.

Excess purine production also occurs in certain forms of anaemia, in leukaemia and in the skin disease psoriasis. A relatively rare cause of gout is a sex-linked genetically determined error of metabolism of the purines.

Symptoms

Gout characteristically comes on suddenly and without warning. The pain is said to be more severe than that of any other form of arthritis. There are several known precipitating factors that bring on an attack of gout. These include:

• minor injury, such as a bump or bruise;

- fatigue;
- worry;
- over-indulgence in food;
- too much alcohol;
- emotional stress;
- sudden starvation or excessive dieting;
- surgical or dental operations;
- serious medical conditions.

The disease usually begins with excruciating pain in and inflammation of the innermost joint of the big toe. This often occurs at night. Other joints may, less frequently, herald the disease – the ankle, the knee joint, a joint in the foot, hand, wrist or, least often, elbow. The affected joint is swollen, hot, red or purplish, and the skin over it is tense and shiny. As a rule, the trouble starts with a single joint, but in later attacks more than one joint may be involved, either simultaneously or one after the other. There is commonly fever, shivering and a feeling of general upset.

The initial attacks usually last for only a few days, but as the disease becomes fully established, attacks tend to last longer. If untreated, they last for days or weeks before eventually subsiding. Some people have one attack only, or attacks at intervals of years. More commonly, attacks are recurrent, with increasing frequency until the condition is constantly present. Full investigation to establish the cause is important.

Gout should never be allowed to go on without proper treatment, because with recurrent attacks the affected joints become progressively more damaged. The results are increasing limitation of movement and joint deformity.

Diagnosis of gout

The clinical features, as described, are so characteristic that the disease is usually fairly obvious. A serious mistake, however, is to assume that you have gout when, in fact, you have a septic arthritis – infection in a joint (see Chapter 7). The moral is that you should never delay seeking medical advice if you have an acutely painful and obviously inflamed joint. Medically, the diagnosis of gout is fairly simple. A sample of blood will show an obvious rise in the uric acid level, and a sample of synovial fluid from the joint, examined under the microscope, will show the typical long crystals. Sampling joint fluid is also an excellent way of distinguishing gout from an infected joint.

Sampling joint fluid sounds alarming, but it is not as bad as it sounds and can be done almost painlessly. There is not much difference, from your point of view, between this procedure and the obtaining of a blood sample. A fine needle on a syringe is passed into the joint and a small quantity of fluid is sucked out.

Complications

It is not to be expected that urate crystals can be deposited in various parts of the body, other than the joints, without causing trouble. The kidneys are among the organs most affected in this way. In Britain, five per cent of all detected kidney stones are formed from uric acid. (This pales into insignificance compared to the situation in Israel, where 40 per cent of kidney stones are so formed, and no less than 75 per cent of people with gout develop kidney stones.) It is also important to know that non-urate kidney stones are 30 times more common in people with gout and high uric acid levels than in people not suffering from gout.

The danger of stone formation in all cases increases considerably if the body is allowed to become short of water (dehydrated). Remember that considerable quantities of water can be lost in sweating in hot weather. A large fluid intake is mandatory for people with gout.

Urate crystals can have an even more devastating effect on the kidneys in some cases. In dehydration and in conditions of high purine production – as when a person with gout is being treated with anti-cancer drugs that kill many cells – crystals can form throughout the whole structure of both kidneys, blocking the tubules and causing complete kidney failure. This is not a common event, but it is, of course, very serious. People suffering it will have to be maintained on an artificial kidney (dialysis machine) until, hopefully, the kidneys recover function. This kind of kidney failure is entirely preventable if there is an adequate throughput of water, so remember always drink plenty if you are a gout sufferer.

Treatment

Advances in treatment now make it possible for most people found for the first time to have gout to live a normal life. The mainstay of treatment of acute attacks is to deal with the inflammation with non-steroidal anti-inflammatory drugs (NSAIDs) such as indomethacin

(Indocid) or naproxen (Naprosyn, Nycopren, Synflex). These are used at the earliest possible stage, and are continued with until the attack subsides and for a week or so afterwards.

Once the affected person is completely free from symptoms, attention is turned to prevention of further crystal deposition, and the removal of urate deposits, by lowering the uric acid levels in the blood and body fluids. This is done with drugs such as allopurinol (Zyloric), which interferes with the conversion of purines to uric acid, or with drugs such as probenecid (Benemid) or sulphinpyrazone (Anturan), both of which promote the more rapid excretion of uric acid by the kidneys. Allopurinol also corrects any tendency for the body to produce excess purines.

The drug colchicine, derived from autumn crocus, is highly effective in treating acute attacks and in preventing further attacks, but it must be used with caution as it may cause side effects. It is prone to cause abdominal pain, vomiting and diarrhoea, and can damage the kidneys and the blood-forming tissues. Large doses can cause paralysis. For these reasons colchicine, once the principal treatment for gout, is now usually kept in reserve and prescribed only by specialists.

Everyone suffering from gout should ensure a high fluid intake of at least three litres a day. This is especially important if there is a known tendency to form kidney stones.

7

Infection in the joints – septic arthritis

Infection is not a common cause of arthritis. This is fortunate, because untreated infection is very damaging to joints. Surgeons have always been very wary of the risk of infection within joints – so much so that for a long time it was considered impossible safely to open a joint surgically. When joint surgery began to get under way, surgeons took exceptional precautions against infection. One pioneer even had a sterile tent set up inside the operating theatre, and worked almost completely enclosed in sterile clothing.

So the first and most important point to be made in this context is that if you have any suspicion that you might have a joint infection, you must not delay getting proper medical treatment.

Septic arthritis affects children and elderly people more than others. As a rule, only one joint is involved, but sometimes several joints become infected at the same time. The most common joints to develop septic arthritis are the weight-bearing joints, especially the knees.

Causes

Any organism capable of causing infection can infect a joint. This means viruses, bacteria or fungi. Germs get to the joint either through the blood or by way of a penetrating injury that enters the joint. The synovial membrane (see Chapter 1) has a very good blood supply, so if there are any germs in the bloodstream there is a possibility that they may land in the membrane. Once there, they soon multiply, set up colonies and, of course, spread into the synovial fluid – and from there to all parts of the interior of the joint.

Happily, it is rare for there to be significant numbers of germs in the blood. That would be the condition of blood poisoning (septicaemia), and the affected person would be obviously ill and fevered. A few germs can, however, get into the blood without causing such dramatic effects, especially if there are infections elsewhere in the body. Another common cause of germs in the bloodstream is intravenous drug abuse. Septic arthritis is rare in healthy people who lead healthy lives, but is much commoner in people whose immune systems are, for any reason, working at less than full efficiency. It is relatively common in AIDS, in people on anti-cancer treatment, and in those with long-term serious illnesses. Anaemia, diabetes and chronic alcoholism also predispose to septic arthritis. People with rheumatoid arthritis or with persistently inflamed joints from other causes are especially susceptible to septic arthritis.

Germs that can cause septic arthritis include a wide range of bacteria, such as those causing pimples, boils, abscesses, sore throats, pneumonia, impetigo, pelvic infection, gonorrhoea and chlamydial infection; and many viruses, including those that cause mumps, German measles (rubella), hepatitis B and AIDS. Less acute arthritis may be caused by *Mycobacterium tuberculosis* – the germ that causes TB – or by various fungi.

When bacteria multiply in a joint they produce chemical activators (enzymes) that help them to get around and to spread the infection. It is these enzymes that do the real damage, because they are specifically capable of breaking down protein, and they quickly attack the collagen protein of the bearing surfaces (articular cartilages). Once this has happened damage is considerable, and it is too late to hope for a complete cure.

Symptoms

The trouble starts fairly quickly, with pain and inflammation rapidly becoming more severe over the course of a few days. Any movement of the affected joint is very painful, so the joint is deliberately prevented from moving. If movement is tried, the normal range will be found to be reduced. The joint is swollen from increased fluid, and is obviously hot. Any pressure on it causes pain. Once the infection is well established, the skin over the joint will usually be red. In most cases there is at least some degree of fever, but this may be absent.

Diagnosis

This may be difficult, especially in people with an infection in a joint already known to be arthritic, but doctors are aware that when any suspicion of joint infection has been aroused, the diagnosis must be established or denied without delay. In any such case, therefore, the prime procedure is once again to take a sample of synovial fluid. In cases of bacterial infection the fluid will be thickened and purulent, and its appearance will add to the probability that the diagnosis of septic arthritis is correct.

The diagnosis will be clinched by the finding of germs. If present, these will always be obtained in the fluid, and can be seen by microscopic examination after staining. It is not usually possible to determine the exact nature of the organisms by inspection, but part of the sample can be cultured on a plate for identification. The presence of large numbers of organisms, however, is enough to establish the general diagnosis of septic arthritis, and antibiotic treatment can be started at once without waiting for the result of the culture. If, after a day or two, the culture and antibiotic sensitivity tests suggest that a more effective antibiotic could be used, the treatment can be changed. The joint fluid obtained will also be examined in the laboratory for its cell content, chemical composition and crystal content (see Chapter 6). In fungal infections, microscopic examination will reveal the typical appearance of fungal strands or buds.

Incidentally, removal of some of the joint fluid is important for a reason other than diagnosis, essential though that may be. It helps by removing at least a proportion of the damaging enzymes, by removing joint debris and by reducing the pressure of fluid in the joint. Even after the diagnosis has been confirmed, it is very common, as part of the treatment, to remove fluid from the affected joint once a day or even more often.

Another important part of the diagnostic process is to look for possible sources of infection. The doctor will therefore carefully check the skin, the throat and nose, the ears, the chest and abdomen, and will enquire into the possibility of sexually-transmitted disease. Samples of urine and stool and, if appropriate, sputum, will be taken. It is routine, in such cases, to take blood to be set up in culture, to see whether any organisms can be grown.

Treatment

This is a hospital matter and requires the attention of an expert. Because of the pain on movement, it is common to rest an infected joint in a splint for a short time. Prolonged splintage, however, is most undesirable if full mobility of the joint is to be restored. As soon as the affected person can bear it, physiotherapy is started to ensure that the joint is put through the maximum range of movement. This is done to prevent fixation in a permanently bent position (flexion contracture), stiffness and weakness in the muscles that move the joint.

The most urgent immediate requirement, however, is to combat the infection by killing the germs. Antibiotics will have been given in large dosage (by injection into a muscle or a vein), even before the infecting organism has been identified. The oral route is not considered sufficiently reliable in this condition. Much relief of the pain can be achieved by regular removal, with syringe and needle, of as much synovial fluid as possible. The joint may also be washed out with sterile salt solution (saline). This helps to remove germs, enzymes and debris, and to keep down the pain. Removal of pus from the joint is considered so important that, if there is little sign of improvement over a week of intensive antibiotic treatment, an operation to open and drain the joint is likely to be recommended.

Because of the synovial membrane's excellent blood supply, antibiotics by intramuscular or intravenous injection will produce an adequate level in the joint, making it unnecessary to inject antibiotics directly into the joint itself. It is, in fact, undesirable to do so as most antibiotics are considerably irritating and can cause a chemical inflammation in a joint. Recovery is assessed by observation of the fluid withdrawn from the joint, which will gradually become clearer and decrease in volume. The temperature will return to normal and the movement at the joint become progressively less painful. Even after all symptoms and signs of inflammation have settled the antibiotics are continued for at least two weeks.

Success depends more on the speed with which the condition is diagnosed and treated than on anything else. If delay allows the articular cartilages to be badly damaged by bacterial enzyme action, full recovery cannot be expected, and a permanently disabled joint or joints will result.

Joint infections from tuberculosis or fungi are less acute and of much slower onset than bacterial infections. They are, quite often, unsuspected for a time, especially if the joint concerned is already arthritic. They are quite rare in the indigenous population of Britain, but are extremely common in the third world and are not infrequently found in immigrants. Again, such infections are more likely to occur in people with immune deficiency from any cause, or in intravenous drug abusers. Effective drugs to combat joint tubercular and fungal joint infections are available. This is not so in the case of most viral joint infections, but many of these will settle if general anti-inflammatory measures are taken.

8

Other rheumatic disorders and problems around the joints

Tenosynovitis

Tendons have sheaths within which they can move freely. The inside of the sheaths are lined with a layer of synovial membrane (see Chapter 1), which provides the necessary lubrication. Tenosynovitis is an occupational disease featuring inflammation of the synovial membrane of a tendon sheath, usually due to overuse. It affects tennis and badminton players, amateur house painters, typists and others who engage in repetitive tasks that put undue strain on tendons. The most common tendon sheaths to be affected are those of the forearm. The tendons of the muscles that extend the thumb are especially prone to tenosynovitis when these are exposed to unaccustomed use.

The condition causes pain in the forearm or other muscles, swelling, and a grating or creaking sensation on movement of the tendon in its sheath – in some cases it is even possible to hear a grating sound. The overlying skin is often red and warm. There is often some limitation of movement, and sometimes adhesions form between the tendon and its sheath, leading to persistent restriction. If the condition is neglected, there will be progressive thickening caused by swelling of the tendon sheath, which may eventually prevent the tendon from being able to move smoothly within the sheath. When this affects the thumb extensor tendons it is known as de Quervain's disease.

Another manifestation of tenosynovitis is trigger finger. In this case, the inflammation involves a tendon sheath, in the palm of the hand, of one or more of the tendons that bend the fingers. Thickening of the sheath does not prevent the finger from bending, but may retain it in the bent position so that it resembles the trigger of a handgun.

Treatment of tenosynovitis is by rest, using either a splint or a plaster cast to provide full immobilization for a time, and the use of anti-inflammatory drugs, such as NSAIDs, or even corticosteroids injected around the affected tendon. Steroids are the most powerful anti-inflammatory drugs available, and are highly effective. Occasionally it may be necessary to resort to surgical freeing of an adherent or over-tight tendon. Rarely, tenosynovitis is caused by infection following an injury. This is much more serious than non-infective cases, and is liable to cause considerable disability unless effectively treated by surgical drainage and antibiotics.

Tennis elbow

At the lower end of the upper bone of the arm, the humerus, are two bumps, one on each side, called epicondyles. Inflammation of the epicondyle on the inner or rear side is called medial epicondylitis, popularly known as tennis elbow. This occurs because several muscles that bend the wrist are attached by a short tendon to this bony bump, and overuse of these muscles causes the attachment site to become inflamed.

Overuse most commonly occurs in tennis by serving with a racket that is too heavy or has too high string tension or is not properly used. The problem may also be caused because the muscles concerned are not sufficiently developed. Other causes include carrying a heavy weight for too long, throwing the javelin, and over-enthusiastic throwing of a ball. Pain is felt at the bony site when the wrist is bent against resistance or when the fist is tightly clenched. If the activity is persisted in after pain has started, the tendon can be pulled partly off the bone, causing real trouble and a prolonged recovery time.

Treatment consists of avoiding any activity that brings on the pain until the inflammation has settled. Re-training is then necessary, under the guidance of an expert knowledgeable in sports medicine. This is directed at performing the desired action by applying force from the shoulder and wrist. Exercises will be necessary to strengthen all the arm muscles.

Musician's overuse syndrome

This is another problem brought on by excessive and repetitive use of certain muscles, and by repetitive light impact. It is usually caused by an increase in the work-load of playing or practising, and is liable to occur in young, ambitious musicians who push themselves too hard. Competition in music is so fierce that many young players drive themselves into overuse. The result is pain and loss of function in the upper limb muscles in pianists and string players, or, in the case of wind players, in the muscles of the lips, cheeks, soft palate or throat. The pain may be severe and disabling, and there is often swelling over the affected muscles and sometimes some loss of sensation. The pain does not necessarily occur at the time of overuse – it may come on hours after a musical session, and can wake the musician at night. It may spread to muscles not primarily involved in the musical activity. Associated with the pain is loss of accuracy, agility and speed, the resulting degradation of technical ability naturally leading to anxiety and depression.

The plain truth is that muscles cannot continue to be used indefinitely without harm, and continuous hard sessions of longer than about half an hour are undesirable. A five-minute break every half hour will allow the muscles time to recover, so avoiding damage. If this regime is neglected, the overuse syndrome is liable to develop, and then much more stringent restrictions become necessary if permanent trouble is to be avoided. Any activity that causes pain must be stopped immediately, even if this means, initially, that periods of playing must be limited to about five minutes. Players should, if possible, avoid other activities that use the affected muscles. In some cases, a radical rest programme, lasting for weeks or months, may be required, and resumption of playing must be very gradual and progressive.

The overuse syndrome is sometimes related to the lack of proper support for the instrument. Supporting posts for clarinets and body-mounted supports for violins and violas may allow musicians to continue to play comfortably.

Repetitive strain injury

Although this condition has become remarkably common in recent years, in 1993 it was actually decreed by a learned judge in a British law court to be non-existent. The paradox arises from a matter of definition. If repetitive strain injury (RSI) is claimed to be different from any of the other known conditions that cause hand and arm pain, stiffness and the inability to perform a particular function, then it is almost necessary to suggest that it is of psychological origin. If the symptoms and disability are caused by inflammation in tendons or tendon sheaths (tenosynovitis) as a result of overuse, or by muscle fatigue, then we know what the trouble is and there is no need to call it RSI.

But people who find themselves unable to continue with a particular occupation because of forearm pain and stiffness are unlikely to be satisfied with the comments of one expert:

'. . . the gigantic and costly epidemic called repetitive strain injury

... can be seen as a complex psychosocial phenomenon with elements of mass hysteria that was superimposed on a base of widespread discomfort, fatigue and morbidity. The epidemic, to which the medical and legal professions, management, unions, governments and media have all contributed, is now waning, but endemic work-related musculoskeletal syndromes remain.'

In fact the epidemic appears to have risen roughly in proportion to the rise in the use of computer keyboards, and interest in it has been much promoted by employment unions concerned for the well-being of their members. However, people with the condition that corresponds to the usual definition of RSI are really suffering not so much from a rheumatic disorder as from what is called a dystonia – a kind of constant tightness in the muscles that prevents them from working properly and causes pain and stiffness. Of course, full investigation by an orthopaedic specialist is required before a diagnosis of RSI is made. If you are deemed to suffer from it, you should perhaps consider whether you are really suited to the occupation causing the symptoms. If this is a matter of economic necessity, it may be worth considering whether you have any underlying and correctable factors, such as a deep anxiety about using computers.

Writer's cramp is a similar dystonia. It is a strange condition, in that it affects only the activity of writing and does not occur when the same muscles are used for other purposes. Soon after starting writing, the muscles involved in holding the pen or pencil go into a state of spasm, as a result of which writing cannot continue. Here too the implication is that there is a psychological element in the causation, possibly related to an unwise or unsuitable choice of occupation. Now that most writers use word processors rather than pens, it is possible that those who develop RSI are those who would otherwise have suffered from writer's cramp.

Carpal tunnel syndrome

This is not actually a rheumatic disorder, but it is included here because it is a common complication of rheumatoid arthritis, and will be of interest to anyone with that disorder.

Most of the movements of the fingers are brought about by muscles in the forearm that have long, fine tendons running across the wrist into the hand. To prevent these tendons from springing away from the front of the wrist when the wrist is bent, a strong strap of fibrous tissues runs over them, forming a tunnel known as the carpal tunnel. One of the nerves running through this tunnel into the hand is the median nerve, and if things get too tight under the strap this nerve may be severely compressed. This is called the carpal tunnel syndrome, and it comes about as a result of swelling due to overuse, local injury, infection or inflammation associated with rheumatoid arthritis. The syndrome can also occur in diabetes, pregnancy, thyroid underactivity and a few other conditions.

The condition is quite common, affecting as many as one person in five hundred. It is especially common in people whose work involves regular repetitive wrist movements, especially with the wrist in an awkward position. Jobs requiring the regular use of force with the hand are liable to cause it, as is the regular use of vibrating tools.

The first indication is tingling and pain in the palm on the thumb side, followed by numbness in this area. These symptoms are made worse by bending the wrist to the maximum degree, and can be brought on by tapping with the finger over the centre of the front of the wrist. The diagnosis can be confirmed by electrical tests of the conduction in the median nerve, which is usually done if treatment by surgery is contemplated.

There is really only one definitive way of curing this condition, and that is by cutting the fibrous strap that forms the roof of the carpal tunnel. When this is done, the medial nerve is often found to be deeply indented by pressure. Surprisingly, no tendon disability results from cutting the strap.

Bursitis

A bursa is a small fibrous sac or bag lined with synovial membrane and normally containing a little synovial fluid. Bursas are located over bony points at which friction or pressure is applied from the outside or from the tendons or muscles passing over them. They make movement easier and protect against undue external force. Bursitis, as you have probably guessed from the name, is inflammation of a bursa. Most cases affect the shoulder region, but bursitis also occurs at the elbow (e.g. miner's elbow), in front of the knee (e.g. housemaid's knee), behind the heel, over the side of the big toe (bunion), over the bones under the buttocks (e.g. tailor's bottom) and so on.

Not all cases of bursitis are caused by undue pressure. Some result from repetitive overuse, some from gout (see Chapter 6), some from infection (see Chapter 7), some from rheumatoid arthritis (see Chapter 5). In many cases the cause remains mysterious.

Shoulder bursitis starts with shoulder pain that is worse on raising the arm sideways. This causes severe limitation of movement of the arm. There is also pain on pressure (tenderness) in certain areas around the shoulder. Often there is visible swelling and redness. In other areas, bursitis produces similar symptoms. The bursa in front of the kneecap can become conspicuously swollen and inflamed in bursitis, as can the bursa over the point of the elbow. Acute attacks of bursitis usually last for only a few days, but can go on for weeks. Neglected bursitis is apt to become permanent (chronic), and the resulting limitation of movement may lead to secondary weakness of muscles from disuse.

Treatment is directed at relieving inflammation, and involves initial immobilization by splintage to rest the affected part for a short period and, at the same time, the intensive use of anti-inflammatory drugs of the NSAID group. Ibuprofen, indomethacin or naproxen are commonly used. If the bursa is greatly swollen from excess production of synovial fluid, some of the fluid can be withdrawn through a sterile needle. A highly effective remedy is to remove excess fluid and inject a steroid drug mixed with a local anaesthetic. This will immediately relieve the pain and will quickly bring the inflammation under control. Before doing this, the doctor must be sure that no infection is present. As the pain settles, progressive voluntary movement is undertaken. In the case of shoulder bursitis, a helpful exercise is to allow the arm to swing in various directions, gradually increasing the angle.

It is a general rule in managing rheumatic disorders that every effort must be made to maintain both the maximum range of joint movement and the maximum muscle power. Exercises are thus an essential part of the treatment, and ideally they should be done under the close supervision of a trained physiotherapist.

Ankylosing spondylitis

This distressing disorder is sometimes called Marie-Strümpell Disease. It is a long-term inflammation of the joints of the spine, the joints between the spine and the ribs, and those between the central and outer bones of the pelvis – the sacroiliac joints. This inflammation leads to a gradual stiffening up and eventual healing over of the joints, so that movement at them becomes impossible.

Ankylosing spondylitis affects men more often than women, and usually starts in the 20s. Nearly all the people affected have the same tissue type – one of the body cell equivalents of the blood groups. The first indication is usually pain and stiffness in the lower back or hip. This is at its worst on rising in the morning, then settles, only to return in the late afternoon or evening. Gradually, the mobility of the spine decreases, as does the maximum chest expansion, which is soon reduced to less than 5 cm (2 in.). The inflammation especially affects the disc area between the bodies of the spinal bones (vertebrae), and as the process continues, the spine becomes more and more solid.

Treatment of ankylosing spondylitis is directed at maintaining joint movement and general mobility, and avoiding deformity. It is most important not to allow fixation to occur with the spine greatly bent. Unless effective management, including controlled exercising and rest, is achieved, there is a risk that the affected person may end up with his chin on his chest. This serious condition, as well as being painful, interferes with vision to the front and with safe walking. In such cases, surgery to remove a wedge from the back of the spine, so allowing a degree of straightening, may be justified. Pain and inflammation can be controlled with non-steroidal anti-inflammatory drugs (NSAIDs).

Cervical spondylosis

This is a disorder of the upper part of the spine – the part in the neck. Degenerative changes occur in the discs between the vertebrae, and bony outgrowths, called osteophytes, develop at the edges of the vertebrae. If you bear in mind that the spinal cord – which is an extension of the brain – runs down through a series of holes in the spine, it will be clear that any new bony growths in this restricted area are liable to cause trouble. They can narrow the canal for the cord, as well as the holes through which the spinal nerves emerge from the cord.

Compression of the spinal cord is a serious matter, causing interference with the conduction of nerve impulses down from, and up to, the brain. This can affect muscle function and sensation. There may be severe pain in the neck, weakness and atrophy of the arm muscles, and loss of sensation in the arms. It may even cause difficulty in walking. The osteophytes are readily visible on X-ray, as is the narrowing of the spinal canal.

Treatment includes the use of a collar to limit neck movement, anti-inflammatory drugs, pulling (traction) on the upper spine and, in severe cases, surgery to remove the bony outgrowths.

Rotator cuff syndrome

The rotator cuff at the shoulder consists of four muscles that normally hold the hemi-spherical head of the upper arm bone (humerus) firmly against the shallow cup on the side of the shoulder-blade in which it moves. Rotator cuff syndrome is the condition in which the tendons of these muscles have become torn or inflamed from repetitive activities requiring the arm to be moved repeatedly above the head. It is thus common in swimmers, tennis players, weight-lifters and people engaged in a variety of other athletic sports. Swimmers doing the crawl and butterfly strokes are especially liable to suffer this disorder.

The condition involves inflammation of the tendons and of the adjacent bursas. To begin with, the pain is felt only when the arm is moved above the head and is brought forward against resistance. Later, pain may occur when the arm is moved forward in a lowered position or when used to push against resistance in a normal position. If the exercise is persisted in, in spite of the pain, there is a danger that the tendons of the rotator cuff muscles may be pulled off the bone.

The condition is treated by initial rest and by exercises to strengthen the unaffected muscles of the shoulder. All movements that cause pain must be avoided. Anti-inflammatory drugs are helpful. If spontaneous recovery does not occur, or if the tendons are badly torn, surgery may be necessary.

Lyme disease

This is a comparatively new disease caused by a recently discovered spiral organism (spirochaete), *Borrelia burgdorferi*, transmitted from animal to humans by tiny Ixodes ticks. The primary hosts for the spirochaete include deer, dogs, mice and other mammals. The name comes from the small community of Lyme, Connecticut, USA, where the disease was first found. It is now known to occur all over the world, wherever Ixodes ticks are found. Ixodes ticks are found all over Britain, and are most numerous in forests and woodland areas where deer are plentiful. The reason this condition is included in this book is that if it is not recognized and treated, a very severe and damaging arthritis may result, among other unpleasant complications.

Infected ticks are acquired in spring and summer, and cause bites through which the spirochaete passes. Over the next month the spirochaetes spread throughout the body by way of the bloodstream. On the skin they produce a highly characteristic sign – a small, raised, red spot, often at the site of a bite, that gradually expands into a ring that may reach 50 cm in diameter. Soon many other rings appear at other sites, and not just the sites of tick bites. The rings are usually on the trunk, buttocks, thighs and armpits, and on the upper parts of the limbs. They usually last for a few weeks, and it is during this time that treatment must be given if the serious late complications are to be avoided. In addition to the rings there are flu-like symptoms – fever, headache, aches and pains, feelings of sickness and tiredness and sometimes painful joints.

Fully established arthritis is rare at this stage, but if the condition is not recognized and treated it will start within a few weeks of the onset in about half the people with the disease. Often the interval is longer – perhaps as long as two years. There is recurrent swelling and pain in one or two large joints, especially the knees, which goes on for several years. Knees that are affected are often less painful than the considerable degree of swelling would suggest, and although commonly hot, they are seldom red. If synovial membrane from affected joints of people with Lyme disease is examined, it is found to be indistinguishable from that of people with rheumatoid arthritis (see Chapter 5).

Treatment with antibiotics such as doxycycline (Vibramycin), tetracycline (Achromycin, Sustamycin) or amoxicillin (Amoxil, Amoram, Galenamox) that kill the spirochaetes is highly effective if given in the early weeks of the disease – the earlier the better. Even in the late stages, antibiotics are helpful and are always used, but the longer the delay, the worse the outlook for the arthritis. If arthritis persists in spite of intensive antibiotic treatment, surgery may be necessary.

Polymyalgia rheumatica

'Myalgia' means muscle pain and 'poly-' means many, so the name of this strange disorder is really just a description of the symptoms. Polymyalgia rheumatica affects people over 50, women about three times as often as men, and causes severe muscle pain and great stiffness, especially in the shoulders, neck, back and arms. The stiffness is at its worst on waking or after sitting for a long time, and may be so severe that the affected person has great difficulty getting out of bed. Women with this disorder describe how they get their husbands to pull them out of bed, or if they are alone, how they first make their way to the edge of the bed by a snake-like wriggling manoeuvre, and then get out by a controlled fall. The most important thing about the disease, however, is that it is associated with another, more dangerous condition called giant cell arteritis (see below).

Polymyalgia often starts suddenly – in the course of a week – and may follow a flu-like illness. It starts with moderate fever, a feeling of being unwell, loss of appetite and weight loss. But the first thing you may notice is that you feel extraordinarily stiff after waking up one morning. Medical examination usually shows that there is a degree of anaemia, but that is about all – the condition is remarkable for the absence of organic signs. There is no genuine muscle weakness, and if the muscles are wasted, this occurs only because the stiffness prevents them from being properly exercised. Muscle samples (biopsies) show no abnormality on examination, and the blood tests for muscle enzymes, which are released when muscles are damaged, are also negative. Electrical tests of the muscles (electromyograms) are also normal. Tests for rheumatoid arthritis and antibodies to DNA are negative.

The one constant and significant feature is that the rate at which the red cells of the blood settle in a tube – the blood sedimentation rate (ESR) – is very high, often over 100 mm of settling in the hour (the normal ESR is less than 10 mm in the hour). When a short segment of an artery is removed for examination as a biopsy, about 40 per cent of people with polymyalgia are found to have an obstructive arterial disease known as giant cell arteritis. This is a dangerous condition because people with it are at risk of suddenly going blind, especially if the arteries on the temples are inflamed and tender. This is very important information for anyone with polymyalgia, because if the ESR is raised, the vision can always be saved by the urgent administration of a large dose of steroids.

Sudden blindness from giant cell arteritis is due to blockage at the end-branches of the main arteries to the eyes (the ophthalmic arteries), but this does not usually occur until after some weeks or months of various local symptoms. These are so important that anyone with polymyalgia rheumatica should be aware of them. They include:

- short periods of loss of vision (known as amaurosis fugax);

- double vision;
- headache;
- pain on chewing.

The headache is increasingly severe, is often at its worst in the areas of the affected arteries, persists through the day and is worse at night. Pain on chewing, known as 'jaw claudication', is a very suggestive symptom – in any patient over 50, it warrants an urgent ESR test.

Polymyalgia is treated with steroid drugs, such as prednisolone (Deltacortril, Prednesol, Predsol) – indeed, the response to steroid treatment is so striking as almost to confirm the diagnosis. A small daily maintenance dose of steroids produces dramatic relief of stiffness and disability, and the treatment is continued for periods of up to two years, after which it is tapered off. If temporal arteritis (arteritis of the temples) is suspected, much larger doses of steroids are given immediately to prevent blindness.

9

General treatments for rheumatic disorders

The effective management of rheumatic disorders calls for a holistic approach. Nearly all the disorders will, of course, require specific drug treatment, both local and general, which has been detailed in the appropriate sections. But in addition to drug treatment, there are several other important measures. These include:

- advice and information on self-help;
- a range of physical treatments, including hydrotherapy;
- occupational therapy;
- psychological counselling;
- complementary techniques for pain relief;
- aids and appliances.

Holistic medicine as a movement has arisen as a reaction to the way doctors' preoccupation with medical technology tends to exclude human factors and relationships. A system that manages patients in a depersonalized way, treating them merely as machines to be modified by drugs, is neither desirable nor particularly effective. The doctor's function is not simply to treat a diseased organ, but to regard the patient as a whole person with feelings, attitudes, fears and prejudices – a person whose needs vary with his or her educational, cultural and environmental background. The best doctors have always practised holistic medicine, but it is important, in this mechanistic age, to remind ourselves of what this means.

The rheumatic disorders are not simply joint, muscle, tendon and ligament problems. They are disturbances of the whole individual, often with implications far beyond the structures that are damaged by the disease. Pain and disability can seriously affect quality of life, often depriving the affected person of activities and pursuits that make life worth living. However charitable we may be, and however deeply we may regret it, there is a primitive reaction within many of us that causes us secretly to look down on people who are disabled. People with disabilities are well aware of this reaction, as a result of which their self-view or even self-regard may be adversely affected.

There is, of course, a strong social movement against discrimination of this kind, but the fact remains that it is present in society. An important part of the holistic management of severe arthritic disorders, therefore, is to do whatever is possible to prevent people from coming to accept, for themselves, this derogatory view. One way of tackling this is to encourage people with rheumatic disorders to accept as much responsibility as possible for the management of their own treatment.

Self-help

The essential thing to remember is that rheumatic disorders discourage you from taking enough exercise. This is one of the main ways in which serious disability arises. Lack of exercise leads to weakened muscles and to a reduction in the range of movement at joints. So you should adopt enthusiastically whatever form of exercise is possible and appropriate to your condition.

What you need are non-impact types of exercise. Among the most useful and valuable of these are swimming, cycling and walking. The object in all exercising should be the dual one of maintaining muscle power and ensuring that, while avoiding pain, your joints are put through the maximum range compatible.

If you are overweight, getting your weight down is also essential – reducing the load on your affected joints will always reduce the severity of your symptoms. Although the principles of weight loss are easy to understand, actually losing weight is never easy in practice, and cannot be done without the unpleasantness of hunger. You must:

- weigh yourself every day;
- cut out all fatty foods, including butter, margarine and full-cream milk in your tea;
- avoid frying – grill or boil instead;
- cut out all puddings;
- never eat ice-cream;
- concentrate on taking carbohydrates in the form of vegetables and fruit;
- use low-calorie salad dressings to make your vegetable dishes more palatable;
- eat fish and white meat rather than red meat.

There is growing evidence that dietary fish oils, especially from oily fish like mackerel, are of general value in rheumatic disorders.

Weight control will also make you look better and feel better about yourself, and may enable you to take more exercise.

Physical treatments

Physiotherapists will be your principal source of advice and practical help in avoiding deformity and maintaining strength, flexibility and range of joint movement. The effectiveness of your physiotherapy will not depend on the lavishness of the equipment in the physiotherapy department, but on the knowledge, enthusiasm, experience, maturity and sympathy of the physiotherapists working with you, and on the quality of the surgical and physical medicine supervision of the physiotherapists.

An effective physiotherapist will be concerned with any factors that affect your motivation, either positively or negatively. They will see to it that you want to succeed, and will give you every encouragement. Try to establish a good relationship with your physiotherapist, and show that you are anxious to improve.

Hydrotherapy is used extensively by physiotherapists. This simply means the use of a small swimming pool, not primarily for swimming, but to relieve the body of gravitational forces so that movement is easier – the natural buoyancy of the body allows movement that may be impossible on dry land. In this way, muscles that cannot be actively exercised in any other way may begin to acquire strength. After a few sessions in the pool, you may well find that you can begin to take over and start to manage your own exercising.

Occupational therapy

This is no longer just a device to keep patients quiet and out of the way of the ward sister. Occupational therapy is now a highly trained and skilled profession run by people who take degrees in the subject. The central concern of people with severe rheumatic problems is not so much pain as their inability to do the things they want to do. This limitation in activity is frustrating and distressing, and greatly reduces quality of life for many people. Occupational therapists make use of purposeful activity to help such people overcome their problems, or learn to deal with them as effectively as possible, prevent further disability and achieve the maximum degree of independence.

To achieve this they must, of course, work in close cooperation with rheumatologists or other medically qualified people, and must be well informed about the nature of the conditions from which their patients are suffering. It is essential for the therapist to be aware of the kind of activity that could be harmful to the sufferer at the various stages of the disorder, but it is equally essential for them to be aware of what is permissible and desirable and that can be helpful. Although the initial concern is to help affected people to cope with the problems that the rheumatic disorder causes in normal daily living, this is not the only aim. The idea is also to maximize functional activity either in the type of activity the affected person wishes to pursue or, if this is impossible, to show and encourage the person to take up an activity that is within his or her capacity.

The first task of the occupational therapist is to make a detailed assessment of the nature and degree of disability and of the person's needs. If these are such as to make normal daily living difficult, the therapist will, at first, concentrate on improving the skills associated with day-to-day activities such as dressing, personal grooming and eating. This might, for instance, involve the use of a model bedroom, kitchen and bathroom, in which the necessary skills may be practised. If necessary, the therapist will draw attention to the existence of the wide range of special domestic equipment that can greatly ease routine household tasks (see below). Many domestic and other activities that are quite impossible to the unaided rheumatic sufferer become relatively easy using such equipment. In some cases the therapist may even be able to develop new methods customized to the patient's requirements. It goes without saying that occupational therapists must also be skilled psychologists.

Psychological counselling

Few people realize how intimately the mind and the body are associated. It is a common mistake to assume that serious bodily changes can occur with little or no effect on the state of the mind. In fact, every bodily change is reflected, to a greater or lesser degree, in changes in the mind, and these changes are often more serious than the physical disability. The commonest effect of a severe limitation in activity is depression, which in turn can so severely affect motivation that the final degree of disablement is much worse than it need be.

In many cases, all necessary psychological counselling can be provided by a sensitive occupational therapist or by an experienced social worker, but there are circumstances in which nothing short of professional psychiatric assistance will do. These are cases in which the reactions of the affected person to the loss of bodily function (and perhaps appearance) are preventing him or her from facing up courageously and effectively to the problem. These reactions, which often involve trying to place the blame for what has happened on others, are called psychological defence mechanisms – they are ways in which we protect ourselves against fully acknowledging events too painful to bear.

Psychiatrists and social psychologists work with patients as individuals or in groups, helping them to understand these reactions, gradually come to terms with the situation, and develop attitudes to the rheumatic problems that are as healthy and positive as the circumstances allow. They help people to adapt to changing abilities and to form new and more appropriate mental attitudes to the changed bodily state. In cases of clinical depression induced by acquired disability, psychiatrists are able to do a great deal by the judicious prescription of antidepressant drugs.

Complementary methods of pain relief

In recent years, pain control has become a speciality in its own right. Pain is a sensation caused by strong stimulation of some of the nerves that carry information to the brain. It is usually a warning that a part of our body is being damaged or is liable to be damaged. Unless very persistent (chronic), it serves as a warning of danger. This is valuable in acute situations, usually leading us to take action to remove the cause of the damage.

But the chronic pain so often characteristic of long-term rheumatic disorders serves no useful purpose whatsoever, and should be controlled. Pain causes distress and anxiety, and is demoralizing and debilitating. If the cause is obscure, it may cause considerable fear. Often these psychological effects are more distressing than the pain itself – pain is less upsetting if the cause is known, and many people stoically endure it because they know and accept the cause and think that nothing can be done about it. This is not necessarily a good idea. If pain is separated from its mental reaction, as is possible by the use of strong pain-killing drugs, it will still be felt, even though it may no longer be particularly unpleasant.

Experts on pain control emphasize that it should be treated by the simplest and safest means available, but that attempts should always be made to relieve it once the cause is clearly known. Pain should be controlled as early as possible; neglected pain becomes more difficult to control. In fact pain-controlling drugs work best if they are used as soon as the pain appears, and should not be withheld until it becomes unbearable. Moreover, different forms of pain control, used in combination, are more effective than methods used in isolation. Authoritative reassurance by a doctor, when appropriate, can also increase the effectiveness of pain-control measures.

The nerves for pain are stimulated into sending pain messages to the brain by the chemical action on them of powerfully irritating substances released from local tissues damaged by the injury causing the pain. Pain impulses can also arise when these nerves are stimulated at a point nearer the nervous system that the actual remote point of the source of the pain. Although the nerves carrying pain impulses terminate in the brain, the pain is usually felt in the region in which the nerve endings are situated.

Nerve impulses passing to the brain may be blocked by local anaesthetics, by electrical stimulation applied to the nerves through the skin, by acupuncture and by the blocking action of other nerve fibres coming down from the brain. Pain is also blocked naturally by substances called endorphins – morphine-like substances produced by the body in response to injury, especially in acutely traumatic emergency situations.

Pain impulses running up the nerve fibres in the spinal cord to the brain have to pass through the equivalent of electronic 'gates' that can be open or shut. These gates are controlled by secondary nerve impulses coming from elsewhere – this is how it is possible to control pain by alternative physical methods such as electrical stimulation of the skin using a variety of machines, skin rubbing with a soft cloth, acupuncture or acupressure, massage or cold sprays to the skin. A popular method of electrical pain control is the TENS (trans-cutaneous electrical nerve stimulation) system. These machines produce high-frequency, low-voltage electrical fields, and are completely safe. The field interferes with the passage of pain impulses in the spinal cord.

Local anaesthetic injections around sensory nerves can completely abolish pain by temporarily paralysing the action of these nerves. The effect is to produce numbness in the area connected to the nerve in question. As soon as the effect of the drug wears off, the nerve will resume its function and the pain will return. But this is not a practicable method of pain control, and it is seldom used. It may, however, be helpful as a preliminary trial before resorting, in extreme cases, to permanent nerve destruction by alcohol injection or by surgical severance. In general, surgical methods of pain control are avoided. They inevitably involve unpleasant permanent loss of sensation and, even when the pain fibres are cut in the spinal cord, do not necessarily succeed in controlling the pain.

It is often supposed that the only useful drugs for pain are the pain-killers. This is not so. Because the mental aspects of pain are at least as important as the physical, drugs that help to control the state of mind in chronic pain can be very useful. A 1997 article in the *British Medical Journal* shows how antidepressant drugs, used to supplement the effect of pain-killers, can make a world of difference to people with chronic pain. The drug amitryptyline is recommended. A small dose, taken at night before retiring to bed, can be highly effective, and only about one person in thirty has to stop taking the drug because of side effects such as dry mouth and drowsiness.

Aids and appliances

Knowledge and effective use of the wide range of aids and appliances available to sufferers form such an important part of coping success-fully with rheumatism and arthritis that a separate part of the book has been devoted to them – see Chapter 11.

10

The radical solution – surgery

Arthroscopy

Although this term literally means 'looking at a joint', the procedure it describes amounts to looking *inside* a joint. Modern arthroscopes are fine instruments that are passed into joints through the skin under local anaesthetic. They enable far more than mere inspection, however, because once the surgeon can see into the joint, other very fine instruments can also be passed in so that surgery can be performed under direct vision. The arthroscope is essentially an ultra-miniature TV camera and bright light source, and what the camera sees is shown on a high-resolution monitor. Surgeons are becoming quite accustomed, these days, to operating without seeing their hands, or even the instruments they are using, directly.

Arthroscopy is used mainly on the knee. The advantages of arthroscopic surgery include a much shorter post-operative recovery period, less pain and discomfort, less scarring, a low complication rate, and often an improved surgical result. The instruments, which include high-speed mechanical cutters and cannulas (small tubes) to flood and expand the joint with sterile fluid, are only a few millimetres in diameter, and leave hardly any scars.

Obviously, the range of surgery that can be performed in this way is limited, and does not include such things as total joint replacement (see below). Although arthroscopic surgery is mainly used for injury cases, especially to remove torn semilunar cartilages in the knee, in selected cases the method is extremely valuable for the treatment of arthritic joints.

It allows a precise evaluation of the state of the joint, and makes it easy to do a thorough wash-out. Therapeutic lavage, as the surgeons call it, results in improvement in over 80 per cent of patients, an improvement that may last for years. People whose knees lock find their condition greatly improved by removal of the offending loose particles. The procedure is of less value in cases in which the joint has become severely degenerate, but partial removal of the synovial membrane (synovectomy), together with a general cleaning up of the inside of the joint, can certainly be helpful.

Synovectomy

This can be usefully performed in conditions in which the synovial membrane has become overgrown and unduly thickened, as can occur in rheumatoid arthritis, haemophilia and a number of rare joint disorders. Formerly, synovectomy was done through a large open incision, but today arthroscopic synovectomy (see above) is the method of choice. Synovectomy is often carried out in cases of rheumatoid arthritis of the knee where medical treatment has failed to produce an adequate response and where there is persistent synovial membrane inflammation (synovitis).

In haemophilia – the hereditary bleeding disorder in which bleeding occurs into the joints, causing great pain and disability – there is often synovitis, in which case synovectomy can be very helpful.

Total joint replacement

Joint replacement surgery is one of the triumphs of modern treatment for severe rheumatic disorders. The results are remarkable. This revolution in treatment began in the early 1960s with the pioneering work of the British orthopaedic surgeon Sir John Charnley (1911–82). Total hip replacement is now one of the most commonly performed operations, carried out when adequate relief of pain or restoration of function cannot be achieved by any other means. It is a major procedure, not to be embarked on casually, and anyone having a hip replacement must be fully informed of the risks as well as the benefits.

Hip replacement surgery

A great many hip joint replacement operations are done because of degeneration of the head of the thigh bone (femur) as a result of fracture of the neck of the bone due to osteoporosis. This causes loss of blood supply to the ball of the joint, which softens, crumbles and dies – a condition known as avascular necrosis. The ideal treatment for avascular necrosis of the head of the femur is to remove the neck and head and replace them with an artificial joint. So far as this book is concerned, however, the great indication for the operation is osteo-arthritis (see Chapter 4). The object of hip joint replacement is to restore a severely disabled person to full mobility.

The operation is performed under general anaesthetic. If you are scheduled for this kind of surgery, you will have considerable pre-operative checks to ensure that there is no infection in your body that might lead to infection of the operation site, the main reason for operative failure. You will also probably be given antibiotics before and after the operation, and your blood group will be checked and some blood cross-matched and set aside in case you need a transfusion during or after surgery.

Hip joint operations are conducted in an ultra-clean environment. Some surgeons operate in special, tent-like modules in which the filtered and purified air supply is kept under positive pressure, and the surgeon and assistants may wear impermeable gowns fitted with exhaust systems to cope with perspiration. Sterile rubber gloves are always worn. These precautions were instituted by Charnley, and contributed much to the success of his early work.

Different surgeons tackle this major procedure in different ways – your incision may be at the front, side or back of the hip. The position you are placed in on the table will depend on the surgeon's approach. The site of the incision and the area of skin well around it is painted with antiseptic fluid, and sterile towels are applied and fixed in place with clips so that only the area of the incision is left uncovered. When the incision has been made, and all bleeding points tied off or closed with the electric cautery, the bone, which lies close under the skin, is exposed.

The surgeon now cuts off the head of the femur, using an oscillating power saw or a two-handled wire saw (a Gigli saw). The bony socket in the side of the pelvis is reamed out to accommodate the artificial cup, and cleared of all cartilage and soft tissue. Keying holes for the cement are drilled into the pelvis, and the cup can now be cemented into place using a thick acrylic cement. The shaft of the thigh bone is now reamed and cleared of all loose and spongy bone, and the femoral part of the artificial joint is pushed down the shaft. The ball is tried in the cup (several of these femoral parts may have to be tried until a satisfactory joint position is found). A wad is now pushed down the hollow shaft to prevent cement from trickling down inside, and the selected part can be cemented into the shaft of the bone and held still until the cement has cured. The ball is now pushed into the cup and the incision stitched up. The operation may take anything from two to five hours.

Infection can threaten the success of the operation, but there is another complication that can actually threaten the life of the patient. The most serious complication of any major procedure on the lower limbs, such as hip or knee replacement, is the formation of large, loose, snaky blood clots in the large veins of the leg. These deep vein thromboses, as they are called, are liable to break loose and be carried up to the heart – and from there to the main arteries of the lungs, often with fatal results. Pulmonary embolism, as this is called, is the principal fear of all surgeons performing these operations, and every precaution is taken to avoid it. Factors associated with high risk of this outcome include an age of over 60 years, a previous history of deep vein thrombosis, concurrent cancer, and obesity. Every person undergoing major joint replacement surgery should be aware of this risk and of what can be done to minimize it.

Preventive measures include:

- promotion of early walking;
- encouragement of movement while in bed;
- the use of graded tension elastic stockings;
- boots that apply intermittent compression to the feet and legs;
- the use of anticoagulant drugs;
- filters inserted into the main vein of the body.

Anticoagulant drugs such as heparin or dicoumarol may be dangerous in people with major liver disease, blood diseases or a history of bleeding peptic ulcer. The use of filters in the main vein (the vena cava) sounds alarming, but they can be placed by way of a fine tube under X-ray guidance, and effectively prevent dangerous pulmonary embolism. They do not, of course, prevent clot formation in the leg veins, but do prevent loose clots from getting to the heart and lungs. Deep vein thrombosis can be detected by ultrasound examination of the veins, which many surgeons arrange for routinely.

In general, the results of total hip joint replacement are excellent. Joints currently being inserted are expected to give at least 20 years of good service. The main complications arise from loosening of the attachment of the two parts of the artificial joint to the bones, or from infection. Re-operation is sometimes necessary.

Knee replacement surgery

The indications for this operation are the same as for hip replacement – pain and disability that cannot be corrected by non-surgical means. Knee joint replacement surgery was slower to get under way than hip surgery, partly because the mechanics of the knee joint were not fully understood. The movements of the knee, including those of the kneecap, are far more complex than simple hinge bending, involving as they do a degree of sliding and rotation. Modern designs of artificial joint take this into account. One orthopaedic team tried out nine different designs of prosthetic knee joint over a period of 13 years. They found that each type had desirable features, but that no one design appeared to offer outstanding advantages over the others. This series of tests, reported in 1985, involved 673 knee joint replacement operations. With gradual improvement in design, however, the results of knee joint replacement became acceptable.

Some of the best modern designs have two parts – one attached to the thigh bone (femur) and one to the main leg bone (tibia) – held in proper relationship to each other using the knee's natural ligaments. This solution provides a very natural knee function, but requires that your ligaments and muscles are in good working order. This requirement, unfortunately, makes it impossible for many people to use this type of prosthetic joint, in which case more complex prosthetic designs will be needed. Success also depends on the surgeon achieving the ideal alignment of the femur with the main bone of the lower leg – the tibia – in both sideways and front-to-back planes. It is essential that the weight axis should pass through the centre of the knee. Guides are used within the shaft of the femur and around the top of the tibia to ensure this. It goes without saying that avoidance of infection is vital.

After the incision is made, the lower end of the femur and the upper surface of the tibia are precisely cut so that their respective artificial components can be set at the correct angle. Holes are then drilled accurately in the two surfaces to fit the stout pegs on these components, and to ensure that the artificial parts fit snugly and tightly. Currently, most prosthetic knee joints are fixed with cement, but trials are still in progress to determine the best methods of fixation (the long-term results of uncemented knee joints are not yet known). The whole operation is likely to take two to three hours, and you may possibly need a blood transfusion, depending on how much blood is lost during surgery.

The length of the recovery period, and the stage at which you start using the knee fully, depend on the type of joint used. What is extremely important is that you cooperate fully with the physiotherapist at this stage, however uncomfortable or even painful the required efforts may be – work at this stage can affect the whole success of the operation. You may have to spend two or three weeks, or even longer, in hospital getting the joint going properly. The physiotherapist may put you on a simple machine that slowly and gently bends and straightens your knee, gradually increasing the range of bending. This is called a passive motion exerciser, but it is not a substitute for your own efforts, and you will have to work to keep your muscles in reasonable shape. The wound stitches will be taken out about two weeks after the operation. This is nothing to worry about.

Satisfactory results are achieved at a follow-up check after ten years in 90 per cent of cases of all knee joint replacements performed by experienced surgeons. Most of the complications can be avoided. Deep vein thrombosis is managed in the same way as with hip replacement operations (see above). It is essential to ensure that the strength of the surrounding muscles and the integrity of the ligaments are maintained over the whole of the post-operative period. The quadriceps muscles on the front of the thigh lose power very rapidly unless regularly exercised, and this exercise must be done, however disinclined you may feel.

Problems are quite often encountered with the artificial kneecap (patella) after joint replacement. This may wear too rapidly on its plastic back surface, or even fracture. Surprisingly, complications involving the kneecap are the most frequent cause of trouble with knee joint replacements. The kneecap lies in the massive tendon that connects the quadriceps muscle to the front of the tibia, and occasionally this tendon may even rupture.

11

Aids and appliances

Self-help devices, and fairly minor adaptations to parts of the home, enable a great many people with severe debilitating arthritis to perform activities essential to normal daily living. You can get all kinds of useful advice and literature from authorities mentioned in the list of useful addresses at the end of the book, but the prime source of advice on self-help and other problems in daily living and occupation should be the doctor or doctors looking after you. You are perfectly entitled to outline your particular difficulties and to ask what can be done to make things easier for you.

You may, for instance, require orthopaedic shoes (or athletic shoes) with good heel and arch support, which can be modified by inserts to meet your individual needs. If, say, the joints between the toe bones and the long bones of your feet are particularly painful in walking, your doctor might agree that a bar – called a metatarsal bar – placed just behind the line of these joints would enable you to bear weight and walk with much less pain. This simple hint can make a considerable difference, especially in people with rheumatoid arthritis.

The association between medical and ergonomic research workers and manufacturers of domestic and paramedical equipment – Boots the Chemist, Chester-Care Ortho Aids, Nottingham Medical Aids Ltd, Homecraft Supplies Ltd, Ortho-Kinetics Inc. and many others – has resulted in the production of a wide range of very useful aids for people limited in their activities by rheumatic disorders. The Arthritis and Rheumatism Council (ARC) can help you find what you need – see 'Useful addresses' at the end of the book. They also publish a free booklet detailing many such aids, written by Dr Barbara Ansell and Sheila Lawton, and there are several larger books on the subject on the market (see 'References and further reading'). Note too that there are Disabled Living Centres, or equivalent establishments, in many towns (a list can be found in the ARC booklet *Your Home and Your Rheumatism*).

General devices

Only a small proportion of what is available to help you can be mentioned in a book of this kind, but here are a few ideas, taken from

ARC literature and elsewhere:

- knives and forks specially designed for people who have difficulty grasping;
- spiked table-top vegetable holders to assist food preparation;
- devices fixed to the wall for gripping the lids of jars so that they can be opened;
- electric can openers;
- electric plugs with large handles for ease of insertion and removal;
- book rests to support books on tables so that the hands can be rested while reading;
- pick-up tongs for retrieving low and high objects without bending or stretching (see section on gardening below);
- various other non-slip gripping devices;
- long-handled dust pans and brushes so you can sweep up without bending;
- lightweight carpet sweepers;
- fitted bed covers;
- duvets instead of blankets;
- tumble-drier washing machines;
- button hooks;
- long-handled shoe horns;
- needle threaders;
- self-opening scissors;
- height-adjustable ironing boards;
- velcro instead of zip fasteners;
- slip-on shoes;
- ready-made ties;
- expandable cuff-links;
- front-fastening clothes, including bras;
- power steering in the car;
- wide-angle driving mirrors to limit the need to twist the body;
- easy-reach seat belts.

Hints for the kitchen

Always try to work at the right height so that you do not have to spend long periods bending down. To achieve this it will usually be easier and cheaper to provide yourself with a suitable high stool or chair, with back support, rather than have the working surfaces raised. Such a chair should also have a bar on which you can rest your feet, and it is helpful to have a solid, movable, box-like step to help you get up onto the chair. If you have to work from a wheelchair, however, it may be necessary to have your kitchen radically altered. Select your fridge with care, bearing in mind the number of times you have to visit it. You may find that a fridge-freezer with the fridge unit on top, or a tabletop fridge, is best.

An extensive working surface is a great help, enabling you to slide equipment around as required rather than having to lift it. Large counter-tops of melamine-covered chipboard are cheap and readily available in do-it-yourself stores, and can often be set on top of existing surfaces to increase the working area. Such surfaces are also easily kept clean if spillages are dealt with promptly.

Sinks can be a problem – often too deep for comfort, and with taps that are hard to turn. It is possible to get sinks no more than six inches deep (about half the usual depth), but you can often make do with a suitable polythene basin perched in the sink on top of an inverted smaller one. You will probably find lever taps much easier to use than standard screw taps, and there are also combination taps that enable you to adjust the temperature by rotating a lever (and the force of the stream by raising the same lever). These taps allow excellent control without having to use your fingers. A cheaper alternative is to get a tap turner lever device that fits loosely over a standard screw tap.

Note that British Gas and the Electricity Council are able to help with the modification of gas and electric cookers, which makes things easier for people with arthritic problems – both produce advice leaflets for disabled people. Consider getting a microwave oven. These are easy to use, quick in action, and easy to keep clean. They are also remarkably cheap. Good accessibility of equipment such as pots and pans, crockery, measuring jars, mixers and so on is important – shelves should be set at the optimum height, and the layout of the kitchen designed with imagination. If carrying trays is a problem, consider getting a trolley with handles for pushing.

Hints for the bathroom

The manufacturers of aids for the disabled have not limited their range to the kitchen. People with severe arthritic disabilities can have a difficult time washing, bathing and using the toilet.

Here special aids are almost indispensable. Handrails can be fitted to a secure surface to assist in getting on and off the toilet and in and out of the bath. It is essential, however, to ensure that handrails are fitted securely, at the correct height, and in the most advantageous position – you alone must judge the last two. Remember that rails can be used either to pull yourself up or to push yourself up. Check by experiment which position is best for you – then get proper professional help fitting the rails.

Non-slip bath seats, of which there are many different kinds, can be a great help. Their advantage is that you need not get right down to the floor of the bath, and they can also make foot washing much easier. You can get combination stool and bath boards, arranged with the stool just outside the bath and the board right across the bath. These too can greatly ease problems getting in and out of the bath. You can even have a good wash while sitting on the board part.

Many people with arthritis find a shower better than a bath, but in either case, the process of overall washing can be greatly eased if properly designed washing equipment is used. Soap on a string; loofahs or sponges with cords; long, scarf-like wash cloths; long-handled body brushes; washing mittens or gloves; and specially designed nail brushes that do not need to be gripped – all these can make a great difference to the ease or even the practicality of the business of washing.

If you have difficulty flushing the toilet, remember that the flush itself can be activated in a variety of ways. A foot-operated flush can be provided if necessary, and in extreme cases, a self-flushing toilet can be fitted. In addition, portable high-level toilet seats that fit over normal toilet seats are available. And there is no need to bid at Christie's for an antique commode! The modern equivalents are smaller, lighter, more convenient, inconspicuous and infinitely cheaper.

Chairs

There is an ARC booklet on choosing easy chairs. It is called *Are You Sitting Comfortably?*, and gives excellent advice on choosing chairs that minimize adverse effects and are easiest to get out of. Unfortunately, not all chair manufacturers are as scrupulous as they might be in their descriptions of their products, many of which are claimed to be 'orthopaedic' and, by implication, suitable for sufferers from rheumatism.

Factors to be considered in selecting a suitable chair include the height of the seat, which should be as high as possible while still allowing you to put your feet, without shoes, flat on the floor. The higher the chair, the easier it is to get out of. The depth and backward slope of the seat are also important. If these are too great the chair may seem comfortable for a time, but is likely to be hard to leave and to provide poor support for your back. A chair should have armrests that are at the right height and that you can easily get hold of. These are also important in enabling you to get up. And a good chair will have a backrest that fully supports your shoulders and your head. If you have serious difficulty in getting out of a chair, you can settle for one with a motorized seat, the back of which tilts upwards at the touch of a button.

Don't take anything on trust. Never buy a chair by mail order that you have no chance to try out before parting with your money. Make the effort to get to the store, and take plenty of time to try out various chairs before making a decision. The most expensive is not necessarily the best for you, but you may have to pay more than you want to get what you need.

Gardening

Gardening is such big business that many tools and gadgets have been developed to make the work easier for the ordinary, able-bodied person. Many of these can also be of help to the disabled person. There are ratchet-action branch cutters with considerable leverage that require remarkably little strength; various grabbers and long-handled weeders capable of one-handed use (some designed to grip and pull out the most stubborn weeds); wheel-rakes that do not have to be lifted in use; ingenious hoes (for example the 'multihoe') that can perform a variety of operations very easily; lightweight lawn shears with long handles for edging and general grass cutting; lightweight wheel-barrows; electric trimmers and hedge cutters – and many other useful gadgets. A visit to the gardening tool section of a large garden centre should pay dividends.

When special gardening aids for people with physical difficulties are taken into account, the actual range of tools available to the disabled gardener becomes even wider. For example, a number of remote gripping tongs, in lengths of four to ten feet, can be obtained for garden tasks, for example fruit picking. And don't forget that tools like these may also come in very handy for general tasks around the house.

If you are severely limited in your activity but still keen on gardening, you might consider a garden in raised pots, or even complete raised flower beds. The latter are available in reinforced concrete, galvanized steel or fibreglass, and come in a wide range of sizes, some with preserved timber exteriors. Seating can be arranged around these raised beds. A herb garden is another possibility.

Glossary

Abduction   A movement outwards from the mid-line of the body or from the central axis of a limb. The opposite, inward, movement is called adduction.

Abrasion   Wearing away of tissue by sustained or heavy friction between surfaces. Abrasion of the biting surfaces of teeth is common. Skin abrasions are among the commonest of all minor injuries.

Acetabulum   The socket in the side of the bony pelvis into which the spherical head of the thigh bone (femur) fits.

Achilles tendon   The prominent tendon just above the heel by means of which the powerful muscles of the calf are attached to the large heel bone. Contraction of the prominent calf muscles pulls the Achilles tendon upwards, so that the ankle is straightened and the heel leaves the ground. The Achilles tendon is essential in walking and running, and is easily strained or torn.

Acromioclavicular joint   The joint between the outer end of the collar-bone and the acromion process on the shoulder-blade.

Acute   Short, sharp and quickly over.

Adduction   A movement towards the mid-line of the body. Muscles that adduct are called adductors.

Adhesion   Abnormal union between body surfaces or other tissues.

Allopurinol   A drug used to treat gout.

Ankylosing spondylitis   A chronic inflammatory disease of the spinal column leading to stiffening and fixity of the ligaments and bones, so that, eventually, almost all movement is lost.

Ankylosis   Fixation and immobilization of a joint by disease that has so damaged the bearing surfaces that the bone ends have been able to fuse permanently together. Sometimes ankylosis is deliberately performed, as a surgical procedure, to relieve pain.

Antibody   A protein substance, called an immunoglobulin, produced by the B group of lymphocytes in response to the presence of an antigen such as a germ. Antibodies are able to neutralize antigens or render them susceptible to destruction in the body.

Antigen   Any substance, organism or foreign material recognized by the immune system of the body as being 'non-self', which will provoke the production of a specific antibody. Antigens include infective viruses, bacteria and fungi, pollen grains and donor tissue.

71

Antinuclear factor　Antibodies directed at elements in the nuclei of cells, such as DNA. Low levels are present in most people, but significantly high levels are found in rheumatoid arthritis.

Antirheumatic　Any treatment for, or prophylaxis against, any form of rheumatism.

Arthralgia　Pain in a joint.

Arthritis　Inflammation in a joint, usually with swelling, redness, pain and restriction of movement.

Arthrodesis　The fusion of the bones on either side of a joint so that no joint movement is possible. This may occur spontaneously, as a result of disease processes, or may be a deliberate surgical act done to relieve pain and improve function.

Arthrography　X-ray examination of a joint after injection of a radio-opaque fluid or a gas.

Arthropathy　Any disease of a joint.

Arthroplasty　The surgical creation of a new joint or the insertion of an artificial joint. Total hip joint replacement is a common example of arthroplasty.

Arthroscopy　Examination of the inside of a joint by an optical device, usually a fine bore fibreoptic endoscope.

Articular　Pertaining to a joint.

Articulation　A joint.

Aspirin　Acetylsalicylic acid. A drug used as a pain-killer, to reduce fever, or as a means of reducing the tendency of blood to clot within the circulation. Aspirin is a prostaglandin inhibitor, which accounts for the wide range of its actions.

Atrophy　Wasting and loss of substance due to cell degeneration and death.

Autoimmune disease　One of a wide range of conditions in which destructive inflammation of various body tissues is caused by antibodies produced because the body has ceased to regard the affected part as 'self'.

Avascular　Lacking blood vessels.

Baker's cyst　A painless swelling occurring behind the knee when there is escape of joint fluid (synovial fluid) through the capsule of the joint as a result of excessive production.

Biopsy　A small sample of tissue taken for microscopic examination so that the nature of a disease can be determined.

Blood sedimentation rate　The rate at which the red cells settle when a column of blood is held vertically in a narrow tube.

Bone　The principal skeletal structural material of the body. Bone consists of a protein (collagen) scaffolding impregnated with calcium and phosphorous salts.

Carpal Pertaining to the wrist or wrist bones (carpals).

Carpal tunnel A restricted space on the front of the wrist, bounded by ligaments, through which pass the tendons that flex the fingers and wrist and one of the two sensory nerves to the hand.

Cartilage Gristle.

Cast A supportive shell of bandage-reinforced plaster of Paris used to immobilize fractures or inflamed joints during healing.

Cervical Pertaining to the neck.

Cervical osteoarthritis A wearing away of the cartilage surfaces of the spinal bones (vertebrae) of the neck. This is commonest in middle age, and causes persistent pain, neck stiffness and sometimes tenderness on pressure over the affected area.

Chondral Pertaining to cartilage.

Chondromalacia patellae A mild form of osteoarthritis affecting the cartilage on the back of the kneecap (patella) and causing pain and stiffness, especially when climbing or descending stairs.

Congenital dislocation of the hip An abnormal relationship, present at birth, of the head of the thigh bone (femur) to the socket (acetabulum) in the pelvis. The condition is commoner in girl babies, and requires early treatment if a severe walking defect is to be avoided.

Coracoid A bony process on the outer side of the shoulder-blade (scapula) that projects forward under the outer end of the collar-bone (clavicle).

Corticosteroid drugs Drugs identical to, or that simulate the actions of, the natural steroid hormones of the outer zone (cortex) of the adrenal glands. Modern synthetic steroids are often many times more powerful than the natural hormones hydrocortisone and corticosterone. They include prednisolone, methylprednisolone, triamcinolone, dexamethasone, betamethasone, deoxycortone and fludrocortisone.

Crutch A portable support, usually in the form of a tubular light metal rod with hand grips and plastic loops for the forearms.

Deformity The state of being misshapen or distorted in body.

Depot injection A drug formulation that allows gradual absorption, over a long period, from a quantity deposited by injection under the skin or in a muscle.

Eburnation The loss or thinning of the bearing cartilage of a joint that occurs in degenerative disease such as osteoarthritis, so that the underlying bone is exposed and becomes dense and polished by friction.

73

Effusion   The collection of fluid in an abnormal site, as in a joint effusion.

Embrocation   Any lotion or medicated liquid applied to the outside of the body in the hope of relieving muscle, joint or tendon pain. Embrocations have little direct effect.

Extra-articular   Outside a joint.

Felty's syndrome   Rheumatoid arthritis associated with enlargement of the spleen and a reduction in the number of white cells in the blood.

Femur   The thigh bone. The upper end of the femur forms a ball and socket joint with the side of the pelvis. The lower end widens to provide the upper bearing surface of the knee joint.

Flexion   The act of bending of a joint or other part or the state of being bent.

Flexor   A muscle that bends (flexes) a joint. A muscle that straightens (extends) a joint is called an extensor.

Frozen shoulder   Painful, persistent stiffness of the shoulder joint that restricts normal movement. The condition affects middle-aged people and usually follows injury or over-enthusiastic exercising.

Gold treatment   The use of gold salts, such as sodium aurothiomalate, to treat rheumatoid arthritis. These are effective in slowing progress of the disease, especially in early cases, but side effects, such as mouth and tongue inflammation, itching, liver and kidney damage and blood disorders, are common.

Gonococcal arthritis   Joint inflammation occurring as a consequence of an infection with gonorrhoea.

Gout   An acute inflammatory joint disorder (arthritis) caused by deposition of monosodium urate monohydrate crystals around joints, tendons and other tissues, especially the innermost joint of the big toe. This occurs when there is excess uric acid in the body, probably as a result of a genetic abnormality. There is excruciating pain and inflammation. Treatment is by non-steroidal anti-inflammatory drugs (NSAIDs) such as indomethacin or naproxen, used early and throughout the attack. Colchicine is also effective. Gout can be prevented by the use of allopurinol, which lowers the levels of uric acid in the blood.

Gouty tophi   Chalky crystalline nodules of a urate salt that may accumulate in the ear cartilage in gout and break through the skin to appear externally.

Haemarthrosis   Blood within a joint space. This can result from injury or disease (such as scurvy or haemophilia). There is pain, heat, swelling and muscle spasm. Such blood is soon absorbed, but repeated episodes cause damage and crippling deformity.

Hallux rigidus   A painful condition in which the joint between the first long foot bone (the metatarsal) and the nearer of the two bones of the great toe is unable to bend properly. This causes severe walking disability. An operation on the tendons may be necessary, or a rocker bar may be fitted to the shoe.

Heberden's nodes   Bony swellings around the furthest joints of the fingers, occurring in osteoarthritis.

Hydrarthrosis   An abnormal accumulation of fluid in a joint.

Hyperextension   'Over-straightening' of a joint beyond its normal limits.

Hyperuricaemia   An abnormally high level of uric acid in the blood. This results in the deposition of crystals of monosodium urate monohydrate in joints and tendons, causing gout. Hyperuricaemia is most commonly due to a genetically determined defect in the excretion of urates by the kidneys.

Interarticular   Situated between articulating joint surfaces.

Intra-articular   Within a joint.

Knee   The sliding hinge articulation between the lower end of the thigh bone (femur) and the upper end of the main lower leg shin bone (tibia). The kneecap (patella) is a flat bone lying within the massive tendon of the thigh muscles, and is not an intrinsic part of the joint.

Latex test   A test for immunoglobulin M (IgM), the rheumatoid factor, in rheumatoid arthritis. Small polystyrene particles coated with human immunoglobulin G (IgG) are clumped in the presence of IgM. The latex test is positive in about 80 per cent of cases of rheumatoid arthritis.

Ligaments   Bundles of a tough, fibrous, elastic protein called collagen that act as binding and supporting materials in the body, especially in and around joints of all kinds. Ligaments are flexible but very strong and, if excessively strained, may pull off a fragment of bone at their attachment.

Lipping   The formation of a curled edge at the bearing joint surface of a bone in osteoarthritis and other degenerative bone diseases.

Loose bodies   Small pieces of bone or of the cartilage bearing surface of joints that have become detached and may interfere with the smooth functioning of the joint. They are a feature of osteoarthritis.

Lyme disease   A disease caused by the spiral organism (spirochaete) *Borrelia burgdorferi*, and transmitted by the bite of the tick *Ixodes dammini* and other species. If untreated it can severely affect the joints.

Mobilization   The process of relieving stiffness or restoring the full range of movement in a joint or a person, usually after illness or injury or after prolonged forced immobility.

Monoarthritis   Inflammation of a single joint.

Muscle biopsy   A method of diagnosis of muscle disorders in which a small sample of muscle is removed for microscopic and sometimes electron microscopic examination.

Myalgia   Muscle pain, especially if persistent and associated with a long-term (chronic) muscle disorder.

Olecranon   The hook-shaped upper end of one of the forearm bones (ulna) that projects behind the elbow joint, fitting into a hollow on the back of the lower end of the upper arm bone (humerus), forming the point of the elbow. The olecranon prevents over-extension of the elbow.

Orthopaedic surgeon   A doctor specializing in the treatment of fractures, dislocations, joint disorders of all kinds, back problems generally, foot bony disorders, congenital defects of the skeleton and many other conditions. Increasingly, the orthopaedic surgeon is concerned with the replacement of damaged and degenerate joints with prosthetic devices, especially artificial hip and knee joints.

Osteoarthritis   A common form of persistent degenerative joint disease involving damage to the cartilaginous bearing surfaces and sometimes widening or remodelling of the ends of the bones involved in the joint. Rheumatoid factor is not present in the blood. Osteoarthritis is an age-related condition, and affects especially those joints that have previously been damaged.

Osteoarthropathy   Any disease involving bones and joints.

Osteochondritis dissecans   An inflammatory disorder of joints in which small fragments of cartilage or bone are released into the interior of the joint, causing swelling, pain and limitation of movement. In some cases loose bodies may have to be removed.

Osteopathy   A system of medical practice that includes many orthodox principles but central to which is the notion that health depends on the proper relationship of the structures of the body to each other. Much emphasis is placed on the importance of the function of the spinal column as a whole, and of the relationship of its component bones to each other and to the pelvis and the limb bones. Osteopathic treatment is manipulative, aimed at freeing and loosening joints and re-establishing proper relationships.

Osteophyte   A bony outgrowth occurring usually adjacent to an area of articular cartilage damage in a joint affected by osteoarthritis. Osteophytes are also common around the intervertebral discs of the spine.

Painful arc syndrome An inflammatory disorder of a tendon or bursa around the shoulder joint, in which pain occurs when the arm is lifted between 45° and 160° from the side of the body. The condition can be relieved by local injections of corticosteroid drugs.

Panarthritis Inflammation of several joints.

Patella The kneecap. The patella is a large triangular bone lying in front of the knee joint within the tendon of the quadriceps femoris group of muscles.

Penicillamine A drug used to treat severe rheumatoid arthritis not responding to non-steroidal anti-inflammatory drugs (NSAIDs).

Polyarthritis Arthritis affecting many joints.

Polymyalgia rheumatica An uncommon disease of the elderly, causing muscle pain and stiffness in the hips, thighs, shoulders and neck. The cause is uncertain. A striking feature is difficulty getting out of bed in the morning. Corticosteroid drugs are effective. Some affected people also suffer from temporal arteritis, and may require urgent treatment with corticosteroid drugs to prevent blindness.

Prednisone A synthetic corticosteroid drug used to reduce inflammation and relieve symptoms in rheumatoid arthritis.

Pseudogout Acute arthritis resulting from the deposition of calcium pyrophosphate dihydrate crystals in a joint. The symptoms are closely similar to those of gout.

Pyarthrosis Severe joint inflammation with pus in the joint fluid.

Rheumatism A common term for pain and stiffness in joints and muscles, as well as for major disorders such as rheumatoid arthritis, osteoarthritis and polymyalgia rheumatica.

Rheumatoid arthritis A general disease affecting women more often than men and, in severe cases, causing progressive joint deformity, joint destruction and disability. The small joints of the fingers and hands are most seriously affected, but the condition can spread to involve the wrists, elbows, shoulders and other joints. Rheumatoid arthritis may also cause loss of appetite and weight, lethargy, muscle and tendon pain, nodules under the skin and severe eye inflammation. There are many complications including joint deformity, instability and dislocation, eye inflammation, heart disease and arterial disorders. Treatment is directed to control of inflammation and complications and the relief of pain by means of rest, splintage, physiotherapy and anti-inflammatory and pain-killing drugs. Immuno-suppressive drugs can be helpful, and penicillamine and gold are also widely used.

Rheumatologist A doctor who specializes in the diagnosis, treatment and total management of the whole range of rheumatic and arthritic disorders. In general, a rheumatologist will be a consultant to whom patients presenting special difficulties are referred by other doctors.

Rheumatology The medical speciality concerned with the causes, disease processes, diagnosis and treatment of diseases affecting the joints, muscles, and connective tissue.

Rose-Waaler test A test for rheumatoid factors in rheumatoid arthritis. Sheep or human red blood cells coated with rabbit antired cell antibody are clumped together (agglutinated) in the presence of rheumatoid factors.

Rotator cuff The tendinous structure around the shoulder joint consisting of the tendons of four adjacent muscles blended with the capsule of the joint. Tearing or degeneration of any of these fibres may cause the common, painful and disabling rotator cuff syndrome, in which there may be inability to raise the arm in a particular direction. Surgical repair may be necessary.

Sacroiliac joints The firm ligamentous junctions between the sides of the sacrum and the two outer bones of the pelvis (iliac bones). Normally the sacroiliac joints are semi-rigid, but in late pregnancy they relax a little to allow easier childbirth.

Sjögren's syndrome An immunological disorder causing reduced secretion of many body glands as a result of damage by antibodies to body tissues (autoantibodies). This causes severe dryness of the eyes, mouth and vagina. The syndrome is commonly associated with other immunological disorders, such as rheumatoid arthritis.

Spondarthritis A group of diseases that feature inflammation of joints, especially of the spine, a tendency to inflammation at tendon attachments, many complications and a negative response to tests for rheumatoid arthritis.

Spondylitis Inflammation of any of the joints between the vertebrae of the spine. This may occur in osteoarthritis, rheumatoid arthritis or, more specifically, in ankylosing spondylitis.

Sprain Stretching or a minor tear of one of the ligaments that hold together the bone ends in a joint, or of the fibres of a joint capsule.

Still's disease Juvenile rheumatoid arthritis. The condition is commonly complicated by the eye disorder uveitis.

Subluxation Partial or incomplete dislocation of a joint.

Synovial membrane The secretory membrane that lies within the capsule of a joint and produces the clear, sticky, lubricating synovial fluid without which smooth joint movement would be impossible. The synovial membrane covers all the internal structures of the joint except the bearing surfaces (the articular cartilages). Also known as the synovium.

Temporomandibular joint   The joint, immediately in front of the ear, between the head of the lower jaw bone (the mandible) and the under side of the temporal bone of the skull. Movement at this joint can often be seen through the skin if the mouth is opened widely.

Temporomandibular joint syndrome   Pain in the side of the face and ear from the effects of spasm of the chewing muscles on the articulation of the jawbone (the temporomandibular joint) lying just in front of the ear. The condition is usually due to emotional tension reflected in muscle contraction.

Tibia   The shin bone, the stronger of the two long bones in the lower leg. The front surface of the tibia lies immediately beneath the skin. Its upper end articulates with the femur (thigh bone) to form the knee joint, and the lower end forms part of the ankle joint. Its companion bone, the fibula, lies on its outer side, and is attached to it by ligaments.

Walking aids   Supports for people with muscle weakness, joint disease or balancing problems. They include plain walking sticks, sticks with three or four small feet, light alloy Zimmer frame 'walkers', elbow crutches and walking calipers.

Water on the knee   A common term for an accumulation of synovial fluid within the knee joint. Such an accumulation is called an effusion, and results from inflammation caused by injury or disease.

Useful addresses

Arthritic Association
Hill House
Little New Street
London W1X 8HB
Tel: 0171 491 0233

Arthritis Care
18 Stephenson Way
London NW1 2HD
Tel: 0171 916 1500
Arthritis Care Free Helpline
Tel: 0800 289170

Arthritis and Rheumatism Council
Copeman House, St Mary's Court
St Mary's Gate
Chesterfield, Derbyshire S41 7TD
Tel: 01246 558033

British Association of Occupational Therapists
6 Marshalsea Road
London SE1 1TV
Tel: 0171 357 6480

Demonstration Aids Centre
The Lodge, Rookwood Hospital
Llandaff, Cardiff
Tel: 01222 566281 ext. 51

Disabled Living Centre
260 Broad Street
Birmingham B1 2HF
Tel: 0121 643 0980

Disabled Living Centre
8 Queen Street
Blackpool, Lancashire
Tel: 01253 21084

Disabled Living Centre
Red Bank House
4 St Chad's Street
Cheetham, Manchester M8 8QA
Tel: 0161 832 3678

Disabled Living Centre
Astley Ainslie Hospital
Grange Loan
Edinburgh EH9 2HL
Tel: 0131 447 6271 ext. 5635

Disabled Living Foundation
Equipment Centre
380–84 Harrow Road
London W9 2HU
Tel: 0171 289 6111

Royal Association for Disability and Rehabilitation (RADAR)
25 Mortimer Street
London W1N 8AB
Tel: 0171 637 5400

References and further reading

Arthritis and Rheumatism Council (ARC) Booklets (see useful addresses). Separate booklets are available on a new knee joint, a new hip joint, ankylosing spondylitis, backache, diet and arthritis, driving and arthritis, gout, guide to choosing easy chairs, introducing arthritis, knee pain in young adults, osteoarthritis of the knee, osteoporosis, painful shoulder, polymyalgia rheumatica, psoriatic arthritis, rheumatoid arthritis, sports injuries, tennis elbow, your home and your rheumatism.

Arthritis in children, *British Medical Journal*, 18 March 1995, p. 728.

Bone loss in rheumatoid arthritis, *Lancet*, 2 July 1994, pp. 3 and 23.

Collagen collagenase and arthritis, *New Scientist*, 8 June 1991, p. 39.

Corney, Richard, *The Carer's Companion*, Winslow Press, Bicester, 1994.

Darnborough, Ann, and Kinrade, Derek, *Directory of Aids for Disabled and Elderly People*, Woodhead-Faulkener, Cambridge, 1986.

Darnborough, Ann, and Kinrade, Derek, *Directory for Disabled People*, Woodhead-Faulkener, Cambridge, 1985.

Disease-modifying drugs in rheumatoid arthritis, *British Medical Journal*, 15 March 1997, p. 766.

Folklore remedies for arthritis, *Pulse*, 14 April 1990, p. 91.

HLA-B27 arthritogenic peptide, *Lancet*, 11 September 1993, pp. 629, 646.

Immunology and joint disease arthritis, *New Scientist*, 4 May 1991, p. 40.

Laryngeal obstruction in rheumatoid arthritis, *British Medical Journal*, 3 February 1996, p. 295.

Lax joints and osteoarthritis, *Lancet*, 5 October 1996, p. 907.

Long-term treatment for rheumatoid arthritis, *Lancet*, 10 February 1996, pp. 43, 347.

Osteoarthritis in old age, *Journal of the Royal Society of Medicine*, September 1995, p. 539.

Osteoarthritis, *British Medical Journal*, 18 February 1995, p. 457.

Osteoarthritis is a genetic disease, *British Medical Journal*, 13 April 1996, p. 940.

Pregnancy clue to rheumatoid arthritis vaccine, *New Scientist*, 24 February 1996, p. 20.

Prolactin and rheumatoid arthritis, *Lancet*, 13 July 1996, p. 106.

Rest or exercise in arthritis? *British Journal of Hospital Medicine*, 21 October 1992, p. 445.

Rheumatoid arthritis – an infectious disease? *British Medical Journal*, 17 July 1991, p. 200.

Rheumatoid arthritis cyclosporin and methotrexate, *New England Journal of Medicine*, 20 July 1995, pp. 37, 183.

Rheumatoid arthritis drug Colloral, *New Scientist*, 14 May 1994, p. 19.

Rheumatoid arthritis drug treatment, *British Journal of Pharmaceutical Practice*, July 1990, p. 236.

Rheumatoid arthritis features and diagnosis, *British Medical Journal*, 4 March 1995, p. 587.

Rheumatoid arthritis management, *British Medical Journal*, 14 August 1993, p. 425.

Rheumatoid arthritis management review, *British Journal of Hospital Medicine*, 1–28 July 1992, p. 106.

Rheumatoid arthritis pathology and management, *Lancet*, 30 January 1993, pp. 283, 286.

Steroids in rheumatoid arthritis, *British Journal of Hospital Medicine*, 6 March 1996, p. 235.

Steroids and joint destruction in rheumatoid arthritis, *New England Journal of Medicine*, 20 July 1995, pp. 142, 183.

Surgical management of the rheumatoid foot, *British Journal of Hospital Medicine*, 6 November 1996, p. 473.

Taping the patella for osteoarthritis of knee, *British Medical Journal*, 19 March 1994, p. 753.

Treating rheumatoid arthritis, *British Medical Journal*, 11 March 1995, p. 652.

Vegetarian diet, fasting and rheumatoid arthritis, *Lancet*, 12 October 1991, p. 899.

Index

INDEX

INDEX